DISCOVER HOW YOU CAN BE THE EXCEPTION AND
START A NEW LEGACY WITH YOUR FAMILY'S HEALTH.

THESE GENES DON'T FIT

JEANNA CRAWFORD

ISBN: 978-1-960136-73-2

This book is dedicated to my baby brother Daniel. You were supposed to be the first published author in the family, not me. Writing this book has shown me a glimpse of what you loved about writing. You will still be a published author. And your writing will minister to those who you ministered to while you were with us. Thanks for all the encouragement.

TABLE OF CONTENTS

INTRODUCTION

Discover how you can be the exception and start a new legacy with your family's health.

This book is for all the ladies who have struggled with their weight and/or blood sugar. Those who have struggled with the guilt, the shame, the fatigue, the disappointment, hiding in pictures or clothes, and regardless of knowing you're beautiful, you just don't feel it.

If you want to lose weight for good, regain your energy, lose that brain fog, and get back into the life that you love this is the book for you.

While our DNA provides a compass for our bodies, it's not a one-way ticket to a certain destination. Yes, our genes play a role. It's our choices that determine the outcome of our body's performance.

Come with me and let's get you back on track. By doing so, you'll be the example to family, friends, and others. Together, we can change the health of our world.

YOU are wonderful!
YOU are beautiful!
YOU are full of life!

Let's get out there and show the world!

CHAPTER 1

CANDY LAND

"Eat less sugar, you are sweet enough already."
—Unknown

I was born in 1971 (I'll save you the math…as of the writing of this book I'm 52 years young), and being a kid in the '70s was a blast! I got to see some of the candy and foods that we know and love today introduced to the food market.

We were healing as a nation—trying to, anyway. Kids were the bright future, a bicentennial was coming up, and it was just a great time to be in America.

While we were in abundance even with gas wars, an oil crisis, and while trying to wrap up a war, income started to rise and kids were seeing the last of the generations that got to run free.

Restaurants were opening quickly. Chains were being established and going up. Gas stations became convenience stores. TV was about to change forever. Cable, music, video games, toys, candy, and great food were all on the horizon.

Just before I was born, Reese's Peanut Butter Cups became so popular that Hershey's had to double production. We all know why, right? Crazy good!

My first adventure with Pop Rocks was at the Tulsa Christmas Parade in 1978, I believe. My neighbors took me and they were like a cool aunt and uncle that loved to spoil me every chance they got. Turns out, that included candy, and I got to enjoy some great stuff.

The caramel- and chocolate-covered cookie pair we've come to know and love as Twix (one of my faves) was actually produced in the United Kingdom in 1967 and finally made its way across the pond in 1979. I remember the first commercial. My mom and I couldn't wait to get our hands on this amazing creation.

Gummi Bears, Big League Chew, and Sour Patch Kids made their appearances in the '80s. We even sent M&M's on the space shuttle that decade.

Dove Chocolate came to us in the '90s, and Hershey Bars celebrated their 100th anniversary and earned the title of the "Great American Chocolate Bar."[1]

When I started kindergarten there was a great board game called Candy Land. You may have heard of it. It's quite possible you've even played it. Milton Bradley released the game in 1948. There's no reading and it requires minimal counting skills so it's great for the littles!! No strategy, only direction. We need to stop right there…NO STRATEGY, ONLY DIRECTION. Take that in for a moment, please.

---

[1] Prince, Jon. "Retro Candy Timeline." *Candy Favorites*,
  https://www.candyfavorites.com/shop/history-american-candy.php

Candy Land is a race. You're playing through a storyline about finding King Kandy, the lost king of Candy Land. You take turns removing a card from the stack and then moving your marker to the next space of the color you pulled on the card. If you draw a named location on your card you have to move to that location, which could be forward or backward. You win when you land on or pass the final square and doing so puts you at the Candy Castle.

Before I get into too much trouble, let me say this: There's nothing wrong with the game Candy Land. The game is not responsible for the sugar epidemic we have today. It teaches kids colors, direction, and how to play with each other. It's quite fun and now comes with a spinner.

My point is this: At a very early age, we introduce and expose our children to candy. If you're anything like me, you grew up with candy. When this game was created in 1948, candy wasn't something that was in every convenience store, at least not in the quantities that it is now. Candy was for special occasions. Christmas, Easter, Valentine's Day, Halloween, possibly birthdays. On those occasions, "a piece or a few pieces" of candy were enjoyed, not entire bags, baskets, or stockings filled with pieces.

According to fooddive.com, consumers spent a record $36.9 billion on candy in 2021. Sweets were used to help us get through the pandemic. Comfort from our childhood, perhaps? People who didn't normally indulge picked up the idea of treating themselves now and then. As adults, there's no one to tell us we've had enough or that we can only have so many pieces. Non-chocolate was the winner in 2021, although chocolate sales did grow, and gum and mints brought up the rear. Maybe it was because we couldn't socialize and weren't concerned with our breath? Food Dive also tells us that despite inflation, candy sales grew to $42.6 billion in 2022. Folks, that's A LOT of candy!!

Ok, so we like candy. What's the big deal, anyway?

I'm glad you asked.

When I was growing up there was a hierarchy to outdoor play. It established what level of "big kid" you were. We started with a tricycle and readily moved that to the side because who didn't want to be cool on a Big Wheel, am I right? Then we couldn't wait to get a bicycle. Then those darn training wheels had to come off! Once you could go past your own cul-de-sac, you've arrived. You can run and ride with your pack and stay out until the streetlights come on.

While the trikes and bikes were active forms of transportation, we walked and ran, too. First of all, not every mom's definition of "be home when the streetlights come on" was the same. Some of us had to run home—and I don't mean a light jog. If you had your bike, you could ride, but you had the obligation to stop and look when crossing the street, and although you did that regardless of whether you were riding, running, or walking, it seemed to go slower on the bike. Hey, we were kids so not all the logic was in place at that time. We ran in our games. We played tag, hide and seek, red rover, red light green light…what I'm saying is that we moved. We moved A LOT!

If candy or sweets were involved in our day it was usually early, unless there was a birthday, wedding, or some sort of occasion, and then we might see something sweet after dinner or in the evening.

Kids' metabolisms were screaming during those years. Walking to school, running to get to class when we were older, sports, outdoor play, games, you name it. Even during pre-teen years, junior high, and high school, how many steps did you get in at the mall? I spent many hours during the day unsupervised with my friends at the mall. Yes, being a '70s kid had its perks, albeit I had to wait until the '80s to enjoy some of that. The bottom line is that movement was a part of our lives.

Unfortunately, during this wonderful time, we also learned that we could have candy, soda, and sweets (cake, snack cakes, etc.) along the way throughout our days. These items were easily accessible in our homes, our friends' homes, at school, the grocery store, and even the gas stations. I'll use myself as an example of how ingrained sugar was in my own life. To this day, I'm still told by those who knew me growing up that it's weird to see me with my water bottle instead of a Dr. Pepper in my hand. I had Dr. Pepper multiple times a day, it was literally part of my identity. I still love Dr. Pepper; I just know now that it's a once-per-quarter (if that) type of thing, and I also know that with one taste the sugar battle is back on for me.

Let's stop here for a minute. Please understand that I had wonderful parents. My friends had wonderful parents. No one knew that we were heading toward a sedentary society, much less a food industry that was going to increase the amount of processed foods and the sugar in those processed foods. No one, other than those in the production industries, saw that coming. I'm not saying those in the production industry were bad either. People want flavor and texture. Sugar provides those things. They were simply trying to sell a product and give consumers what they wanted. Unfortunately, that meant we were hooked on sugar by the time we got to make those decisions and thus became the consumers who craved it.

Our parents:

- Loved us
- Wanted better for us
- Strived to give to us when they could
- Were enjoying the time we were living in

And didn't know what was coming.

Those of us who now have our own children and grandchildren are no different.

I was lucky as a kid. The tech came later so I wasn't as drawn to it. My parents didn't get it so they didn't much care if I was drawn to it or not. I spent a lot of time in the garage with my dad. I'm sure I was a great "help"—at least I thought I was. I got to paint, bring tools, and make sure he had tea (southern sweet tea...I didn't know people drank it without sugar until much later in life) when he was thirsty. I "helped" haul hay. I was little during that phase, but it included some serious play time in the field when we stopped. I'm sure my getting to "help" had something to do with Mom having the house to herself to cook and clean in peace. I'll also never forget playing with kittens, puppies, goats, chickens, and whatever wonderful thing was at Lee's Feed Store when we visited there. And those hay-hauling days and trips to the feed store also included breakfasts of Slim Jims, Twinkies, and Mountain Dew. Soda has been a part of my life since before I could remember.

I had chores (yes, I'm lucky for that). Church activities for kids then were active. My grandparents ran a dairy farm, so those visits were also active, both with work and play. Watching my brothers meant playing with them. Well, mostly playing. We were siblings, we had differences. But I loved that time with my brothers and wouldn't trade it for the world. I also helped my dad roof, helped my mom with the ironing she did on the side, or did the chores and cooked so she could iron and make some extra money during the times she got to be a stay-at-home mom.

Not only would sugar consumption grow in our world later in my childhood, but movement was slowing down. Maybe not so much in my life, but things were changing.

Cable TV—a wonderful world with more than four channels, could it be? Indeed!! Then there was Atari, our beloved first in-home video game system. Bowling alleys, skating rinks, restaurants, and eventually the stand-alone arcade meant that time spent being active was now spent captivated by a screen. Add Play Station, Sega, handheld games, computer games, and the computer itself—and it no longer was the size of an entire wall (What?!? Turns out Gene Roddenberry was a genius!). In fact, computers became smaller and smaller. We carry them in our pockets today, with games!!

Technology had kicked off and it was consuming our lives. While some used portable music to keep moving, others used our tech to sit still and veg out. YouTube wasn't around yet so if you wanted to watch music videos you stayed in front of the TV. Some danced, but a lot of us just sat in amazement, waiting to see what Van Halen, Cyndi Lauper, Ozzy, Pat Benatar, and many others would produce next.

Movies, movies, movies…so many great movies. Again, another sitting activity. Then you could rent them! Now they're in our homes and we're moving even less.

We were becoming still. Sports took a back seat to tech and our movement activities in society became less and less important.

Now, back to Candy Land.

So, the foundation was laid in the land of abundance where we could have and get just about anything we wanted. Our parents guided us, of course they didn't allow us too much. So, what happened by the time we hit college age and became parents ourselves?

Per Zipdo.co, the average American consumes around 77.1 grams of sugar per day. Let's put this in perspective. That's approximately 18 teaspoons of sugar per day. That's 103% more than is recommended, which is 38 grams or 9 teaspoons according to the American Heart Association (Note: Men can have more than women, I didn't break that down to keep it simple. If you want statistics specific to gender, send me a note and let's talk).

So where are we getting all of this sugar from? Because even with those crazy big stats on candy, we're not sitting around eating candy all day long. Remember, we were taught better than that.

The CDC tells us that the leading sources of added sugars (which include sucrose, dextrose, table sugar, syrups, honey, and sugars from concentrated fruit and vegetable juices) are sugar-sweetened beverages, desserts, and sweet snacks. A lot of the rest is coming from processed foods, condiments, cereals, etc.

Fast food has been documented to include extra sugar, salt, and fat to increase flavor in the food. You've seen this in articles, on TV, people have even gone on fast food-only diets to show us. I've seen a drive-through or two or 100 in my years living. Have you? Of course, we all have. It was another part of that evolving society of abundance and being able to have what we want, when we want it, and fast!

Friends, we didn't just find the Candy Castle. We didn't just get acquainted with King Kandy. We befriended the king, moved into his castle, and saturated our lives with sugar. Then we were content with our tech and stopped moving.

But wait, there's more…

Per USDA data on table sugar, there was a drop in consumption from over 90 lbs. per person per year in the early '70s (yes, that says 90 lbs.) to just over 60 lbs. per person today.[2] That sounds good but…

High fructose corn syrup (among other things) came into the picture in the early '70s. Enter "added sugars."

Kids drinks begin having added sweeteners during that time. Folks, that included baby formula.[3]

With high levels of added sugars being introduced at very young ages, we are now seeing two generations carrying higher risks for

---

[2] Bussler, Frederik. "Americans Are Eating Mind-Boggling Amounts of Sugar." *Medium*, 10 Aug 2020, https://medium.com/analytics-vidhya/americans-are-eating-mind-boggling-amounts-of-sugar-f9fd5b4b4d06

[3] "High-Fructose Corn Syrup." *Wikipedia*, https://en.wikipedia.org/wiki/High-fructose_corn_syrup

heart disease, stroke, type 2 diabetes, and certain types of cancer.

Generation X, do I have your attention now? Millennials and Gen Z, please read on. Builders and Baby Boomers, please read on and support new efforts.

Again, while there is someone or something to blame for this, that is not the focus of this book. The blame game gets us nowhere.

What I want you to leave with is this:

This can be turned around.

You don't have to become diabetic or have heart disease, and you can certainly fight off some of those cancer cells by reducing sugar.

Sugar and sweets are not evil. In fact, they are meant to be enjoyed. You can do that. You can't do that all day every day. But I can show you how to enjoy sweets at times and not do your health in.

Now that we know all of this, I'm going to share a quote from my mentor, Darren Hardy: "You are 100% responsible for your life." Let that sink in because we're going to need it later.

CHAPTER 2
MISUNDERSTOOD MESSENGERS

"Your genetics load the gun. Your lifestyle pulls the trigger."
—Dr. Mehemet Oz

Spoiler alert: There are A LOT of stats and data in this chapter. If you'll bear with me here we'll get to the more entertaining part. These stats are important and will lay the necessary foundation for you to make some great health choices for yourself. Your future self will thank you, I promise.

Let's talk about genes for a minute, also referred to as genetics. What is genetics? According to the National Institute of General Medical Sciences, "Genetics is the scientific study of genes and heredity–of how certain qualities or traits are passed from parents to offspring as a result of changes in DNA sequence."[4]

What are the three types of genetic diseases?

Genetic diseases can be categorized into three major groups: single-gene, chromosomal, and multifactorial. Changes in the DNA

---

[4] "Genetics." *National Institute of General Medical Sciences,* 4 April 2022, https://www.nigms.nih.gov/education/fact-sheets/Pages/genetics

sequence of single genes, also known as mutations, cause thousands of diseases.[5]

I get it…snooze…ZZZZZZZ.

Genetics and Diabetes

"Type 1 and type 2 diabetes have different causes, but there are two factors that are important in both. You inherit a predisposition to the disease, then something in your **environment** triggers it.

That's right: genes alone are not enough. One proof of this is identical twins. Identical twins have identical genes. Yet when one twin has type 1 diabetes, the other gets the disease, at most, only *half* the time. When one twin has type 2 diabetes, the other's risk is three in four at most."[6]

"Type 2 diabetes has a stronger link to family history and lineage than type 1, and studies of twins have shown that genetics play a very strong role in the development of type 2 diabetes. Race can also play a role.

Yet it also depends on environmental factors. Lifestyle also influences the development of type 2 diabetes. Obesity tends to run in families, and families often have similar eating and exercise habits.

---

[5] Genetic Alliance; The New York-Mid-Atlantic Consortium for Genetic and Newborn Screening Services. "Understanding Genetics: A New York, Mid-Atlantic Guide for Patients and Health Professionals." *National Center for Biotechnology Information,* 8 July 2009, https://www.ncbi.nlm.nih.gov/books/NBK115568/#

[6] "About Diabetes: Genetics of Diabetes." *American Diabetes Association,* https://diabetes.org/about-diabetes/genetics-diabetes

If you have a family history of type 2 diabetes, it may be difficult to figure out whether your diabetes is due to lifestyle factors or genetics. Most likely it is due to both. However, don't lose heart! Studies show that it is possible to delay or prevent type 2 diabetes by exercising and losing weight."[7]

I started this chapter quoting experts for a reason.

I'm not a genetics expert.

I'm not a doctor.

I'm not a college graduate.

I am smart.

I'm a formerly-diagnosed pre-diabetic.

I lost my mind momentarily when I learned that.

I had a holistic doctor who encouraged me to deal with this naturally and do my research.

I know how to research.

My mom left me a gift when she left this earth—a book called *Beating Cancer with Nutrition,* by Patrick Quillin—that led me not only to this information but to this conclusion. That gift led me to some great doctors who have done some great research.

I became a nutrition coach for a purpose.

My life's mission is to let you know that genetics play a part in type 2 diabetes, but it's not a guarantee that you will or have to

[7] Ibid.

get it. In other words, you do not have to be diabetic just because the disease runs in your family.

"Type 2 diabetes is primarily a dietary-caused disease related to eating processed foods highly prevalent in the Standard American Diet (SAD) and across the modern world today. Excess fat on the body increases insulin resistance leading to diabetes, but other factors that place a biochemical stress on the beta cells in the pancreas that secrete insulin, such as repeated glycemic stress and chemicals, can play a contributory role. Even though the risk of developing type 2 diabetes may be higher if you have others in your family with the disease, it doesn't necessarily mean that you will develop it. Being overweight and eating too many animal products and refined foods is so common today that diabetes is exploding worldwide. Lifestyle changes, which include regular vigorous exercise and a Nutritarian diet-style, are not only preventative but in most cases, they enable patients with this condition to make a complete recovery."[8]

In the previous chapter, I set the stage for you by showing you how the world, the food industry, and we as humans have embraced convenience, taste, texture, and all things "good" for the sake of eating. Our nutritional values have somehow escaped us. Many decisions were made supposedly for good. Many of those decisions were not necessarily good. The SAD (Standard American Diet) has failed us. Even today we've gone past processed foods to GMOs and now to bio-engineered food.

---

[8] "Type 2 Diabetes." *Dr. Fuhrman*, https://www.drfuhrman.com/health-concerns/53/type-2-diabetes

Statistics About Diabetes from the American Diabetes Association website (these numbers are from 2022):[9]

Overall numbers

- **Prevalence:** In 2019, 37.3 million Americans, or 11.3% of the population, had diabetes.
    - Nearly 1.9 million Americans have type 1 diabetes, including about 244,000 children and adolescents.
- **Diagnosed and undiagnosed:** Of the 37.3 million adults with diabetes, 28.7 million were diagnosed, and 8.5 million were undiagnosed.
- **Prevalence in seniors:** The percentage of Americans age 65 and older remains high, at 29.2%, or 15.9 million seniors (diagnosed and undiagnosed).
- **New cases:** 1.4 million Americans are diagnosed with diabetes every year.
- **Prediabetes:** In 2019, 96 million Americans age 18 and older had prediabetes.

Diabetes in youth

- About 283,000 Americans under age 20 are estimated to have diagnosed diabetes, approximately 0.35% of that population.
- In 2014–2015, the annual incidence of diagnosed diabetes in youth was estimated at 18,200 with type 1 diabetes, 5,800 with type 2 diabetes.

---

[9] "About Diabetes: Statistics About Diabetes." *American Diabetes Association*, https://diabetes.org/about-diabetes/statistics/about-diabetes

Diabetes by race/ethnicity

The rates of diagnosed diabetes in adults by race/ethnic background are:

- 14.5% of American Indians/Alaskan Natives
- 12.1% of non-Hispanic blacks
- 11.8% of Hispanics
- 9.5% of Asian Americans
- 7.4% of non-Hispanic whites

The breakdown among Asian Americans:

- 5.6% of Chinese
- 10.4% of Filipinos
- 12.6% of Asian Indians
- 9.9% of other Asian Americans

The breakdown among Hispanic adults:

- 8.3% of Central and South Americans
- 6.5% of Cubans
- 14.4% of Mexican Americans
- 12.4% of Puerto Ricans

Deaths

Diabetes was the seventh leading cause of death in the United States in 2019 based on the 87,647 death certificates in which diabetes was listed as the underlying cause of death. In 2019, diabetes was mentioned as a cause of death in a total of 282,801 certificates.

Cost of diabetes
As of November 2, 2023
$412.9 billion: Total cost of diagnosed diabetes in the United
States in 2022
$306.6 billion was for direct medical costs
$106.3 billion was in indirect costs

After adjusting for population age and sex differences, average medical expenditures among people with diagnosed diabetes were 2.6 times higher than what expenditures would be in the absence of diabetes.

I need for you to see these numbers. You need to feel these numbers. But more than anything, you need to know that you don't have to be part of these numbers. Please note that I'm talking about type 2 diabetes here. Type 1 is something that you are born with, although some aren't diagnosed until later in life.

Can you beat diabetes?

Yes, you can.

Can you beat it if you're already diabetic?

Depending on how far you are into the disease, yes, you can. You will need to involve your doctor. That can be a challenge because not all doctors are equally trained in nutrition. Regardless, you can take nutrition into your own hands, advise your doctor, and have him or her monitor your numbers to adjust medication according to your progress.

What is diabetes anyway?

"It's a chronic (long-lasting) health condition that affects how your body turns food into energy.

Your body breaks down most of the food you eat into sugar (glucose) and releases it into your bloodstream. When your blood sugar goes up, it signals your pancreas to release insulin. Insulin acts like a key to let the blood sugar into your body's cells for use as energy.

With diabetes, your body doesn't make enough insulin or can't use it as well as it should. When there isn't enough insulin or cells stop responding to insulin, too much blood sugar stays in your bloodstream. Over time, that can cause serious health problems, such as heart disease, vision loss, and kidney disease."[10]

If you're not seeing it yet, sugar overtakes your bloodstream. When your blood is full of sugar it can't carry the oxygen and nutrients to parts of your body that need it. It also can't carry away the carbon dioxide and other waste materials to be removed. Your blood is the transport system and if it's altered, your cells start to die off. You can't fight off infection, you can't renew cells, you don't clot properly, and you can't regulate your body temperature. When cells die our health fails.

It's a result of a hormonal imbalance. Once one hormone goes the others follow, like a domino effect. Hormones are the body's messengers. If the messages aren't being delivered, the body can't

---

[10] "What is Diabetes?" *Centers for Disease Control and Prevention,* 5 September 2023, https://www.cdc.gov/diabetes/basics/diabetes.html

function properly. Insulin is a major hormone in the body. If it's out of whack, your body is out of whack, period.

Reducing your risk is important. Here's how:

Maintain a healthy weight or lose weight. Easier said than done, I know. Abdominal fat is key here, you want to lose that. Even a 5 to 10% weight reduction can lower your risk.

Stay active. Aim for 150 minutes per week. Avoid sitting for a long time.

Eat more plants. This is where my studies with Dr. Fuhrman served me well. Fruits, vegetables, legumes, nuts, seeds, and whole grains (you gotta watch the whole grains, folks—read those labels) are essential to reducing your risk for diabetes. Lose the processed, pre-packaged foods where you can.

Know your numbers. Regular maintenance and check-ups are important. You need in-depth lab work. A general screen isn't going to tell you what you need to know. Find a holistic or naturopathic doctor who will dig deep into your bloodwork so you know where you need to start.

Lots of people live with diabetes. Medicine is advancing all the time. However, the best defense to beating diabetes is a good offense. In other words, don't get it. If you do, catch it early while you can still do something about it.

Diabetes causes a high risk of heart attack, stroke, and kidney failure. It can cause permanent vision loss by damaging the blood vessels in your eyes. You can develop problems with your feet from nerve damage and poor blood flow.

This chapter is doom and gloom, I get it. I'd give anything if I could paint a better picture, but I can't. Why am I sharing this? I didn't know a lot of this stuff. I grew up and started raising my own kids thinking I knew what a balanced diet was all about. Sure, I knew soda, cookies, candy, and too many sweets weren't good, but I had no idea the impact that would have on my health. I also had no clue how much sugar was in the food I was eating. Like many, I thought if the FDA thought it was OK to be on the shelf then it was safe to eat.

It's time to wake up, folks.

No, you don't have to give up every sweet thing you love on the food spectrum. You do need to eat or drink it more responsibly.

You don't have to give up meat if you don't want to. You do need to incorporate more plants, seeds, nuts, whole grains, and whole foods into your diet. That's what we were designed to eat and thrive on. Without them, we're in trouble.

What I enjoyed more than anything on my journey back to health was adding rather than taking away. What I learned was that by adding better things I didn't have room, nor did I want the not-so-good stuff. There are always going to be things that if I get a taste the battle is on. Remember that Dr. Pepper I talked about? It gets more manageable over time. In fact, it's simple to get your health back—but it's not easy.

Let's move away from the stats, doom, and gloom and I'll share my story. Hopefully, by sharing, you'll be encouraged to take the steps you need to and keep going until you're living and thriving again. Thank you for reading this far. Your time is valuable and I appreciate your sharing it here with me.

CHAPTER 3

LIFE IS GOING TO HAPPEN

"You alone are responsible for what you do, don't do, and how you respond to what's done to you."
—Darren Hardy

Let me lead with this…while I wasn't happy, entertained, or the least bit grateful in the moment finding out I was pre-diabetic, after some thought (which, believe me, came after a full-blown pity party and temper tantrum—I'm human y'all) and some research, I knew exactly how I got there—and actually, some of that journey was a lot of fun, some was out of my control, and some of it, let's just say I could have responded better. Let me add—I now know how to have a lot of fun without wrecking my hormones, blood pressure, and entire system in the process.

The Mayo Clinic states the risk factors for type 2 diabetes as follows:[11]

---

[11] Mayo Clinic Staff. "Type 2 diabetes." *Mayo Clinic,* 14 March 2023, https://www.mayoclinic.org/diseases-conditions/type-2-diabetes/symptoms-causes/syc-20351193

- Weight
- Fat distribution
- Inactivity
- Family history
- Blood lipid levels
- Age
- Pre-diabetes
- Pregnancy-related risks
- Polycystic ovary syndrome

Johns Hopkins adds:

- Stress

I'm going to address these individually. Some will have little or nothing to do with where I found myself on diagnosis day; others are profound. With that in mind, remember that it doesn't take ALL of the risk factors. Get even a few of them involved and you could be headed down a slippery slope.

Weight

I am the mother of a 34-year-old son and a 33-year-old daughter. I had my son on my 18th birthday and prior to that, I was rarely ever over 110 pounds, and usually hovered around a size 6. Yes, sadly, in high school I thought I was fat.

When I was carrying my son, I gained maybe 25 pounds, and did not show until the last two months of the pregnancy. According to the monitors I was in labor for a while but I only felt 45 minutes of it. Prior to that I worked out with the wrestling team in high school. I didn't want to wrestle on the team, or at all, personally. I was just friends with a lot of the guys, interested in lifting and fitness, and loved having 20 or so "brothers" to hang out with at school. I was young, I was in shape, and my body handled the baby business well and I bounced back quickly.

I was also recently married, had a tiny kitten, was finishing two semesters of high school and was looking to graduate on time and toward the top of my class (which I did by the way) in addition to 25 to 38 hours a week working retail. If you haven't figured it out by now, I'm an overachiever, and that had kicked in in full force by this point in my life. Failure was not an option in my mind. Looking back now, I wish it had been, at least in regard to graduation, the retail job, and a few other minor things. I will say failure was never an option as a mother, and as long as there's breath in my lungs it never will be. My kids are my pride and my joy. I am also a daughter and big sister, which means the world to me. Sadly, I was discovering that although I thought I was a friend to many, only a few stuck with me. While I appreciated those few, the many that fell to the side felt like failure to me. Enter stress over what I thought were failures at this point in my life. To be clear, there were no failures. Perceived stress, good stress, bad stress, it's all stress, folks. Your body does not know the difference.

I had just returned to a size 4 (ish), had a good routine going with my firstborn and my husband had found a good job, albeit without insurance, when I found out I was pregnant with my daughter. My head space, my heart space, my spiritual connection had all been challenged and here come the hormones and another human growing inside me. This was one of those moments in life I wish I had known what was coming down the road. What these kids would become. Who they would become. I was 19 years old, scared, emotional, and had no clue how to handle life much less a marriage, mortgage, and two infants. I had no reason to be scared, it would all work out, but again, youth.

Depression set in after the birth of my daughter. I had some complications from childbirth that made it next to impossible to walk for a while. That actually generated some treasured time with my great aunt who was a tremendous help to me, and we shared some very special times. I got to hear stories about my great-grandmother and how she raised her seven children.

At this point in my life, I packed the weight on, and not just a little bit, either. I did get help for the depression and was on and off meds for about 10 years. If you're having an issue with that and can't control it with exercise or other natural methods, do get help.

When the kids were older, and were in school and after-school activities, I did make a commitment to myself and lost the weight. While I thought I did it in a healthy way, it was only somewhat healthy. Still, best to get the weight off, and I did that, returning to a size 8. Gang, I lost 8 dress sizes! It took work, it took time, and it took getting real creative with my workouts and food, but it can be done.

Fat Distribution

Fortunately for me, my weight gain was proportional from head to toe. I say fortunately because my weight distribution was not the belly fat that is concerning to health. Extra weight is not good, but if you're going to gain, you want to do it all over.

What started my health journey was that I had put on some fluff again. The kids were grown, out of the house, and I had met the man I'm married to now. I got comfortable, I got lazy. Once again, I looked in the mirror, said "Enough," and got back to it. The weight started to come off, but it was slower and harder this time.

One morning I was getting ready for work and noticed that my muscles were not toning back up like they had in years past. Believe me, I was putting in the cardio and the resistance training. Most of me looked good but the muscle tone wasn't there. Then, I noticed my tummy was sticking out more than usual. I've always enjoyed an hourglass figure at any weight and this was gone. I put my hand on my belly and just about lost it. It was as hard as a rock!

A lady that I worked with had been seeing Dr. Charles Edwards in Glenpool, OK, at Revolution Health of Tulsa Functional Medicine. If you are in my area of the world, I highly recommend these folks. She was having some different issues and had gone on about how in-depth they were with blood work. I knew I needed some help so off to this doctor I went. While I was shocked at what I found out, I needed to hear it, and I am still with this doctor to this day. They helped me get my health back. These are the folks who helped me learn that I was pre-diabetic, inflamed, had heart disease markers lit up like Christmas, and my hormones were shot. As in my testosterone came back "non-detectable," shot. That's not good.

A lot of learning, a lot of bloodwork (still), a lot of grit, determination, and literal sweat, and after two years I got my health back. I'm here to tell you, it's worth it. I teach up to four Zumba fitness classes a week, sometimes more; I lift weights, I work a full-time job, and I coach nutrition on the side. To say I'm busy is an understatement but I have the energy and drive to do this because I am healthy. You can be too.

Inactivity

There have been a few periods in my life when I've been inactive. Every single time in my adult life this happens my health takes a hit. I quote Denise Austin a lot: "If you rest, you'll rust." She knows what she's talking about.

I'll tell you this…If you have a family history of or have been found to be genetically predisposed to diabetes or any other heart disease, you will have to keep moving your entire life. Our bodies were designed to move. Our current sedentary lifestyle with our SAD diet is taking out people we love left and right.

You MUST keep moving!

Family History

Being a human like the rest of you, when I first heard I was pre-diabetic I started wondering who in my family was diabetic. I only knew of a few. So, being the smart kid I am, I asked. Whoa!! I had no idea so many people on both sides of my family had it.

I'm not real big on family medical history because too often I've seen my own past doctors take that information and use it to incorrectly diagnose me. While Dr. Edwards asked about it, he didn't draw any conclusions until he had the lab work back to compare the two. What I'm trying to say here is choose your doctor carefully. Of course, your family history has a valid place in your medical records. Just make sure that the work is being done to confirm a diagnosis rather than letting that information determine your path.

Doctors, I mean no disrespect here and that scenario is certainly not across the board. In our world of 15-minute doctor visits, you can see how it would be easy to rely on family history. Patients, your doctor works for you. Work with them, direct them, and you are responsible for your health. If you're not getting what you need or finding answers keep looking. They are there.

The other thing I will tell you is to get with your family and discuss medical history. Many times, we rely on what we can remember. Take it from the goofball who did that for years—it doesn't serve you well. Ask. Write it down. Keep it handy. If you have loved ones who have passed, see if their spouse or children will help you with getting their records if they don't have them already.

One last note on this—let's go back to our genetics chapter. Just because something seems to run in your family doesn't mean you have to get it. The genes determine which direction the cellular breakdown will take. The trigger in your environment is unknown to you. So, if something keeps coming up in family history, look at the causes of that something. It could be that there is heart disease, obesity, diabetes, cancer, etc. due to generations of the family diet and activity. Family history is a tool, not a set-in-stone map for your health. Always remember that.

Blood Lipid Levels

Let's say this in English: We're talking about cholesterol here.

I did not have any issues with cholesterol numbers until the hard fat set in around my belly. However, I also was not having my blood checked regularly so there's no telling how far back this started for me. This is why I tell my clients, KNOW YOUR NUMBERS. Pay attention to them, get your blood checked, see what's going on in there.

After the shock and pity party wore off (y'all I was mad, really mad, and at myself) and I started studying, I learned about the power of plant-based and whole foods. I went 45 days plant-, whole food-, seed-, and nut-based, and my numbers got in line quickly!!

No, I'm not telling you to become a vegetarian. I'm not telling you meat is bad for you. I'm telling you that we do not eat enough plants and we are robbing ourselves of the amazing work they do for our bodies. I do eat meat but not every day. My protein shakes are plant-based. I eat a lot of vegetables now. I've not had one issue with cholesterol since. You can take that information to the blood bank. See what I did there?

Age

Have you ever heard that you can't beat a bad diet by working out? If anything proves that, it's age. We have all met the runner or gym person who says they work out so that they can eat what they want. We've all heard the stories of a runner or recreational athlete who dies suddenly. How can that be? They work out or run all the time. You cannot avoid nutrition folks, you just can't do it. At some point in time, it's going to catch up with you.

The older we get, the more "mileage" our bad habits have on us. Just like interest building in a bank account, years of habits, good or bad, will manifest over time. Get the nutrition right and you'll have lots of years of mileage.

> *"Small, seemingly insignificant steps completed consistently over time will create a radical difference."*
> —Darren Hardy–*The Compound Effect*

The older we are the more habits we'll likely need to correct. The more habits there are to correct, the harder this may seem. But you are never too old to old to start. Don't forget that.

Pre-Diabetes

This is where I landed. This was due to a combination of not being consistent with great choices, sometimes making good choices rather than great ones, and some just flat-out bad decisions. Consistency is key here. Misinformed choices were also part of the equation.

The bottom line is this: I wasn't working out, I wasn't getting nearly enough protein, fruits, or vegetables, I was struggling at best to eliminate sugar from my diet (carb junkie here folks), I was inconsistent with what I did that was healthy (other than water— I've been drinking a gallon a day for over 25 years), and later learned that some of what I thought was healthy really wasn't.

There is SO MUCH information out there. This is why I highly recommend working with a coach and a doctor, checking that bloodwork, finding out what it is that you can do to improve that bloodwork, and continuing to do it.

When I greatly increased my consumption of fruits and vegetables, got moving again, kept the water up, and slowly (I'm not kidding, this takes time, and depending on your upbringing and the food you were raised on THIS IS HARD), ever so slowly, weaning myself from non-whole grain breads, non-whole grain or veggie pasta, soda, etc. I was finally able to start getting my energy, stamina, vitality, and health back. It's a journey. You don't get there overnight and you're not coming out of it overnight.

Pregnancy-Related Risks / Polycystic Ovary Syndrome

I personally cannot speak to these. But, again, I suggest that you seek out a great doctor, get that blood work, find those numbers, and keep them good. In the case of the latter, you are likely going to need multiple doctors. I wish I could be of more help here, but I can't, so I'm going to know in my heart you'll seek out the help you need.

Stress

In case you didn't notice, stress was probably the most consistent piece of my story above. Those two wonderful kids I told you about, I ended up raising them mostly by myself. I did not remarry until they were grown, and one was out of the house and the other was almost out. There were some job changes, multiple relationships, kids in school, kids out of school, graduation, boot camp…if you've been a parent or an adult for any length of time you get the idea. Throw in some moves from house to house in there, will ya? That was some extra spice in my life.

Not all of the stress was bad. Unfortunately, the body does not understand the difference between good stress and bad stress. It's all just stress to the body. Some stress was created, some of it just comes from life.

I have a background in workers' compensation claims and litigation defense, and at the time I wrote this, I was working full-time in Loss Control, which not only includes workers' compensation but also property and casualty, theft, general liability, and catastrophic loss in the heavy highway construction arena. From the time I hit the workers' compensation field, there have been deadlines, court rulings, battles, you name it in front of me. My encounter with every injured person was the result of something bad happening. Yes, I've seen some wonderful outcomes, I've seen good people get back on their feet and I've had some great resolutions for claims in every area mentioned. All of it starts from someone being harmed or wronged, all of it has the potential to become combative, and not all of it ends as intended. It's a tough line of work and I've been doing this for over 35 years now.

Where I fell short in all of this is that I did not have a good stress relief system. During the times in my life when I was consistently working out, I did much better. I can look back now at how I dealt with some tough times and got through them gracefully because I had that release from working out. During the times in my life when I wasn't working out, even the smallest stress moments would unravel me. This was a big factor in my decision to become a fitness instructor. If you're teaching a group fitness class, you have to be there. The workout may not be the same and I don't always have to go full out, but I do have to be there and I do have to move. Let's just say I still have stress, but I handle it much better these days.

I've also learned that pedicures aren't just for pretty toes. It is restorative for very tired feet that single, single double (aka dance)—A LOT! Massages are for tired muscles. Both of these help clear my head. Long walks (strolling here folks, not power walking) clear my mind. Reading in a quiet space clears my head. Writing in a quiet space clears my head. This is a work in progress, but I promise you that if you take some of these techniques or find some of your own you will help yourself greatly.

While stress alone doesn't cause diabetes, there is evidence that there may be a link between stress and the risk of type 2 diabetes. "Stress has long been shown to have major effects on metabolic activity."[12]

If you have any of the risk factors listed here, do yourself a favor: get some stress relief tools, use them, and don't let that be what pushes you over the edge.

---

[12] Surwit, R. "Stress and Diabetes Mellitus." *National Center for Biotechnology Information*, 15 October 1992, https://pubmed.ncbi.nlm.nih.gov/1425110/#

CHAPTER 4

WIPEOUT

(Insert music and crash video here in your mind. Think of the types of videos on *America's Funniest Home Videos* that are funny to us, but not so much to the person who was filmed.)

You've likely heard the saying, "You didn't gain all the weight overnight and therefore you won't lose it overnight." Well, the same applies to becoming type 2 diabetic. With or without knowing it, I went on a journey that landed me there.

I'm going to do my best to recap my journey for you. While yours will be different, if you pick up on any of the same behaviors or events, you might want to really pay attention here.

Here's where I believe this started for me. To be fair, it likely started before this, but here's where my mind goes...

I had a fella in my life, and we had made plans for the future. Let's just say we were informally engaged, shared a house (but not a bedroom), we ate well, took care of ourselves (or so I thought– looking back he was ill or didn't feel well A LOT), wrote Christian music together, and had started looking into how we would serve God together.

Remember when I told you before that I'm human? Well, I had the rose-colored glasses on, friends. The lens that I looked at life through was, shall we say, distorted. I didn't see the writing on the wall. I didn't pay attention to the signs. I made excuses in my head. What I believed was going on was in fact a fabrication of what I wanted to be real.

Long story short, he left abruptly (at least it seemed that way at the time), and it HURT!

The breakup itself was cold and mean. I was devastated. Whether I should have been or not is irrelevant. Looking back, it shouldn't have been that bad. That's how far I'd gone to convince myself that this was the real deal. Sad on my part, yes, but it won't help you or me to hide how I felt at that time, because it started a series of events and choices that I would later pay for. Let me be clear here, that's on me.

At this point in my story, I'd like to share that although we are not "friends," we are cordial; we still share some of the same friends and I still talk with his family. We've even swapped our favorite recipes that we enjoyed together. Many years later, I do not believe for one minute that he ever set out to hurt me. Our lives were going in separate directions, and he spared me a lot of grief and most likely a divorce. I'm explaining something that happened to me. I'm not trying to jab someone or paint a bad picture of him. Are we good here?

Fortunately, I knew enough about dealing with depression, and with this being an actual life event where it would be normal to grieve and feel depressed, I did go to my doctor to get some help there. We went through an exercise in which she had me write down all of the life changes I had been through recently. At the time I didn't appreciate going through this, but with what I know now, it was necessary and brilliant.

My list looked something like this:

- Started dating someone.
- My son (Austin) graduated from high school (if you've never been through a senior year with a kid, you're in for a wild ride. Lots of memories, emotions, celebrations, you name it. It's a great but crazy year).
- My parents, youngest brother Daniel, and I dropped Austin off at boot camp three weeks after graduation.
- Finally found a well-paying job (I had lost my job previously and the replacement was much less than I was making).
- Found out my daughter (Ashlee) was having some life issues.
- Ashlee moved in with her dad. This was her senior year.
- I moved out of my house.
- I had to return my beloved Mastiff, Duchess, to the wonderful people who gave her to me.
- I moved to a different town.
- Ashlee graduated from high school with her class, on time.
- I went through the breakup and moved back to the town where I lived previously all within 72 hours.

I filed for bankruptcy (remember that "failure isn't an option" thing? Yeah, this one hurt).

Folks, this all happened in one year, give or take. Some of these life changes are good. We talked before about the body not knowing the difference between good stress and bad stress. Let's just say that by this point, I was a hot mess.

Let's stop for a minute, please. Do not feel sorry for me. Again, most of these things were the results of choices I had made. My mentor Darren Hardy reminds us that our life, at this moment, is the sum total of all the choices we have made. You'll note on the cover of this book that I ask you to "be the exception" to leave a legacy for your family. That is a phrase he uses regularly and if you're going to "be the exception," your choices have to be the exception. That means you break from the herd mentality and make good choices, the right choices, regardless of what everyone around you is doing.

This is just the base of the groundwork of how I landed in a doctor's office hearing the words "you're pre-diabetic, and this list of other things." I put myself on this path. I accept that and I own that.

The problem isn't that all of this happened. The problem was my response to it.

I quit eating.

I couldn't sleep.

When I did eat, it was fast food or takeout.

I went through the grieving process multiple times.

My focus on anything (other than fishing, oddly enough) was extremely limited.

While those are natural responses to a loss, what's not natural is that I became locked into that pattern for a long time. Much longer than I should have. I've lost my mom and my baby brother and although the pain is still there, and grief still creeps in, I was functional within months rather than over a year. Yes, over a year.

I was malnourished, fatigued, and lost.

Although I wasn't eating right, I did work out some. Not like I do today, but I knew that it would help me with the depression, and it did. On the days that I would hit the gym, my clarity was much better. I was again able to come off of the medication I was taking for my depression.

Other things happened during that time, and like anyone else, some were good, some were bad, and most were the result of my choices. I did start eating again and, as I did before, did what I thought was "healthy." Some of it was, some of it appeared to be, but I've learned A LOT since that time and now know that I could have done better. That's OK. We can't do better until we know better.

There were relationships, some good, some I probably should have done without. My son deployed to Iraq. The day he returned to the States my younger brother deployed to Afghanistan. My son went to college in San Diego after leaving the Marine Corps, and my daughter was finding her place in the world. My knee was injured pretty badly due to a slip on some ice. I met the man who is now my husband. Quit my job to start a consignment business, watched a friend's life fall apart, and began to work on coordinating my grown kids, my husband's kids, and my family.

Life goes on and we have to take care of ourselves as it does.

Just when I thought that things were beginning to calm down in my life the unthinkable happened. My mom got sick. We initially thought it was the flu. She would get better and then worse and then better again. I believe in my heart that she knew what was going on. We had no idea what was coming. My dad called me on a Thursday; Mom's eyes had turned yellow, which we knew was not good at all. She was admitted to the hospital on that Thursday, and by the following Tuesday, the day after Christmas 2012, she was gone.

This was much worse than the pain of the breakup. I was once again hurting and lost. We were close, and I had lost my longest and closest friend. I did keep eating, working out wasn't an option, and worry for my dad had set in. He was capable of taking care of himself, but being the oldest kid, I felt like I needed to be there for him until I was comfortable that he was OK. It was a shorter journey for him than it was for me. That's not a negative reflection on my dad. He was fully capable. I just couldn't deal with losing my mom and focusing on him rather than myself helped me avoid working through my grief. Not a good plan but again, another choice I made.

During the year after my mom's passing, I moved again as things had become serious between Cody (my husband) and me. I was trying to figure out how to run an online business and believe me, was really getting some practice on failing here. That would serve me later in life with my second business, the one that I have now—the one that brought me to you.

I felt like I needed to fill Mom's shoes, keep the family together, and do holidays, meals, and all the things. I tried my best. Not being emotionally ready to take that on or even knowing if I could or should, comfort food became more and more common in my diet. The weight started to pack on.

My dad, months later, met a sweet lady and the Lord blessed him with another to love. She, too, had lost a spouse, and the two of them clicked and were married. Knowing he was OK and moving on, my grief cycle started again. Enter more comfort food.

My injured knee wasn't getting any better. I reopened my claim and began physical therapy in the hopes of finding some relief. I was trying to work out, but it was difficult due to the pain. I knew I had to keep going and did my best to get the work in. While that went on, I was helping my dad sell the house and the land where he and my mom had lived. Clearing things out, going through their things—lots of emotions and memories going on during this time. I had also returned to part-time work, as the online business world had not been as successful as I'd hoped. I kept going because that's who I am and that's what I do.

Still dealing with a knee that would not cooperate, the insurance carrier refused to authorize further physical therapy. I was now looking at the potential of surgery. At the same time, my husband had learned that he had avascular necrosis in his hip joints (yes, both of them) and would undergo having both hips replaced. Due to insurance, deductibles, and timing, this was done right after we moved into our house and eight weeks apart. That's right folks, just long enough to get one working well enough to support the other. As you can imagine, this was very painful for him, and recovery took a while. Six months later I had five procedures done on my knee. One of those included cutting into a bone, tapping it up, and screwing it back down. We were quite a pair during that time!

I didn't realize how painful my surgery and recovery would be. Depression set in and, thankfully, it was circumstantial and only ran its natural course. Unfortunately, comfort food was again the norm and, being unable to walk, much less do anything else, the weight really packed on.

Let's stop here for just a minute, please. Does any of this sound familiar? Job changes, loss of a loved one, medical conditions, surgeries, recoveries, helping family, building relationships, moving? It's life and it's how we react to life. I'm stopping here to remind you that no matter how much you know about nutrition and health, your mind, your emotions, and your circumstances play a role in your decisions. They certainly did with mine. Yes, give yourself some grace during those times. Yes, enjoy some comfort during those times. You just can't stay there. Emotional eating is a real thing. Stress eating—or not eating—is a real thing. If these are moments in time, that's fine. If they are not, get a coach, get some help, see a doctor.

Once I was mobile again, enough was enough with the food and inactivity. It still hurt to walk; running was out of the question. The treadmill hurt but I still did it. In fact, once my claim was over, I did buy a nice treadmill and I put some miles on her. It still wasn't the best activity, but it's what I had. Our pool, for the first time in my life, became a source of exercise. My daughter was taking a new dance fitness class and she raved about it. All I heard from her was Zumba this and Zumba that. I love to dance but growing up I wasn't allowed to and thus wasn't very good at it. She kept inviting me and I kept putting it off. I finally gave in one day and I was hooked; I was TERRIBLE at it, but I was hooked! I knew this was how I was going to literally get my groove back, and I did. I was able to modify the moves until I was strong enough to go full steam ahead. Full steam for me is not necessarily the same as for others, but it felt good to leave 15 lbs. on the dance floor. Fast forward to today, I teach three to four times a week and work out in addition to that.

I kept doing my physical therapy exercises (I do them to this day) and regained strength and mobility in my leg. I did manage to tear the meniscus on my other knee, but thanks to what I learned in the post-op, I was able to rehab myself back from that. So, it was back to business. I went back to work full time. Helped my dad finish moving from the property. It was during this time that I found the gift that my mom had left me, the book called *How to Heal Cancer Through Nutrition* that I mentioned before. This is college-level stuff, a tough read, but so worth the time. I was introduced to many wonderful doctors through this reading. I came across and still follow Dr. Tom O'Bryan and Dr. Joel Furhman. It was through this channel that I came to be acquainted with these two doctors and started to learn some serious things about nutrition and health.

With what I learned in a short time and with my new love for Zumba (I'm a licensed instructor at this point—I got the license for the sole purpose of learning HOW to do Zumba properly), I lost 15 pounds on the dance floor, another eight from changing how I ate. However, I was starting to notice some issues.

I had returned to full-time employment; this is where I landed the Loss Control Manager position at the construction company where I am at the time of writing this. I felt decent, looked good, worked out, and my nutrition was improving. BUT…I was TIRED! My brain was foggy. It was getting to the point that it took everything I had to get through a full day of work. My dancing slowed down or didn't happen at all, and comfort food once again made an entrance.

Our general counsel at work had been working with a holistic doctor on some health issues she'd been having and recommended that I go see them. When she told me they didn't take insurance and it would be a battle to file the claim on my own, I knew I had found a good doctor. That may sound odd to you, but having been in the insurance industry the majority of my career, having a baby brother born with a heart condition and watching how health insurance readily pays for prescriptions well before they'll pay for preventative measures that aren't on their pre-approved list, I knew that this doctor was wise not to let the carriers dictate how he ran his practice. This was one of the best decisions I've ever made. I still see this doctor to this day and if you are in the northeast Oklahoma area, I highly recommend Dr. Chad Edwards at Revolution Health & Wellness. If you are not local, look them up, look at the credentials, treatments, and programs that they offer, and find someone similar in your area: https://Revolutionhealth.org

I went in for an appointment and had a full panel lab done, the results of which are 13 plus pages (this is a legit blood test, gang). Looking back, I feel foolish now, but I honestly thought they were going to tell me my testosterone was low (I had learned just enough to be dangerous at this point), tell me how to treat it, and send me on my way. I could not have been more wrong.

The results come back color coded for a lot of the test fields. Green is good, yellow you may need to pay attention to, and red, obviously, is not where you want to be. To an ADD (self-diagnosed) overachiever it's a thing of beauty from a visual standpoint. When I first saw it, I really expected to see a lot of green. Again, I…WAS…WRONG!

As we started going through the results, I literally felt the color in my face turning as red as the blocks on my chart. I could also feel my blood pressure rising (which was already bordering on high as it was). I was in my mid-forties and was a statistic waiting to happen.

Low testosterone (it actually read "could not detect").

Inflammation markers were high (If you don't already know, that is NOT good).

Heart disease markers were lit up like Christmas.

Thyroid numbers were off.

Blood pressure was borderline high.

I don't even remember the rest, although I do have the report still. I was livid! Not with the doctors, the lab, or the results, but with myself. I knew better. I might not have known then what I do now but surely, I knew better than to be in this position or this shape. I was angry, hurt, disappointed and—I'm going to be honest with you here—it might have taken a long time, but I was dying.

I huffed, I puffed, I stomped, I cried, I threw things, I said bad words, I looked in the mirror and yelled at myself. I cried some more, paced, thought, fought with myself, asked God why (totally not His fault and I knew it—one of those heavenly Father moments—I'm sure He consoled me while He stifled His chuckles like a good parent does), and just shook my head.

This lasted a couple of days. Literally, that's all it was, but I made sure it was a worth-my-while, full-blown adult temper tantrum. But I knew in my heart that I had work to do, and it would come down to that moment of decision. Was I willing to do what it took to figure it out, put that into practice, and save my life? Once I got to that question, I went to sleep. I had changed my question of "why" in my prayers to "show me."

And He did show me. And He led me. And had I not followed His lead I would not be writing this book and sharing with you today.

CHAPTER 5

THE STARTING LINE

I had the data I needed, although I wasn't thrilled about it.

I threw the fit and dealt with the emotions that came with the data.

Now it was time to get started!

Have you ever started looking into:

- Losing weight
- Lowering blood sugar
- Lowering cholesterol

Or reducing inflammation naturally?

The amount of information out there is MIND BLOWING! While the internet is a beautiful, wonderful tool, it over delivers to the point that we get stuck. Too much information will paralyze, confuse, overwhelm, and derail you. And it will do that quickly!

This is where I really had to stop and take a good, hard look at what my goals were and how I was going to get there. Standing still wasn't an option for me. Doing nothing wasn't going to help me out. In fact, I was convinced that every day that I waited was a risk. So, what to do?

I'm not a sit still, do some meditation, find my Zen kind of girl. I think those things are wonderful, I've just not mastered those arts at this point in my life. But I do know that Psalm 46:10 tells us, "Be still, and know that I am God…" I focused on what was in front of me. I listened to what was around me. My heart told me that although I hadn't been diagnosed with cancer, I had a nutrition book in my hands and that was where I needed to start.

They say that when the student is ready, the teacher appears. If you Google the phrase, you'll find it's attributed to multiple authors. Regardless, it's a saying, and it's quite true. Here's why— when you want something, especially nowadays in this techno world we live in, once you search for it you start to see it everywhere! Say you're looking for a new car; you search for a while and land on one that you like. You've chosen the color, interior, wheels maybe, lots of factors. Ads pop up everywhere, in your email, on your social media ads, it's like they're reading your mind! They're not really, they just study your search history. Anyway, you'll also notice that you start to see this car around town. At stop lights, on the highway, in parking lots, you name it. Well, Google is good, but it's not THAT good. Is this some sort of magic? Maybe a connection to the universe? Why is this happening?

You have become aware of a desire. You have focused on that desire. The car that you imagine driving in your future didn't just magically appear everywhere, you just became aware that it was there. It was around this point in my life that I was reminded of this. Any time I have wanted something I started searching and eventually found my way. I knew that this was not going to be any different.

So, my mind calmed and my frantic search ended. I would start with the book and see where this journey took me. I had complete faith that the right path would be there for me to find as I went along, and that's absolutely what happened.

Don't get me wrong, I was still concerned and felt an urgency to correct the wrongs, but I was at peace with the decision.

Why am I sharing this? Have you been to the starting line? Have you approached it, been overwhelmed, and decided that you'll do something later? Are you still there and haven't made a decision (which, by the way, is a decision)? Maybe you've noticed some similarities between my story and yours and you're looking at the starting line for the first time. Perhaps you've been to the starting line, started, and never finished. It's OK. Many others have done that as well.

Let's talk about the Starting Line for a moment because it's a neat place.

You're Not Alone

Have you ever done a 5K or some sort of race? Maybe you've watched them on television or gone to a horse or car race. Everybody starts in the same place.

For our purposes here I'm going to use the foot race analogy to help paint the picture:

It's race day. Tons of people are around. There are competitors and those there to cheer them on. Bigger events have vendors, sponsors, maybe even sports reporters to cover the event. Excitement is in the air. Some people stretch, others jog or find some way to warm up. As start time approaches there's a push in the crowd. Everybody wants to be up front. At that moment, you're literally part of a herd. What's interesting is that most of these races no longer begin all at once. There's no need to start at the same time, as your chip will determine when your clock starts. Still, everyone wants to be up front.

Sound familiar? January 1, New Year's Day, you cannot get a parking space at the grocery store to save your life! Workout clothes at the store? Nope, they're all picked over. Meal prep dishes? Good luck finding those. That's why our Christmas lists look familiar year after year, full of these items so we can shoot out of the gate when the starting gun fires!

Most of us have been there, celebrating New Year's Day in a frenzy of meal prep, new recipes, working out, and explaining to our families that there's a new sheriff in town.

You Have Your Own Pace

The race starts, footsteps are all that can be heard (faint cheering in the background—if you're a runner or participant, it's background noise). The front of the crowd starts to pull away, the entire line of people running or walking is starting to spread out. Your training has kicked in and your pace is set. Some use others to set their pace. Others have their own. Some get lost in the tunes from their headset and let the race unfold.

The same applies to weight loss. Whether you started with the New Year crowd, with a group during the year, or on your own, you will have a pace. Some have a quick pace at first and then slow down. Some will have a steady pace throughout. Others start slow and pick up momentum. I've done all three and I will tell you, I prefer the last one. If you start with one thing, master it, and continue to build good, healthy habits, not only will you lose the weight for good, but you will also do it in a way that allows your body to keep up with the changes and you won't cause yourself other health issues. Remember that good stress/bad stress concept? This applies here. Too many changes at once causes your body to think it's under stress. While you're doing something good for yourself, it's interpreted as stress and your body will fight back. Slow and steady really does win this race, folks.

The Finish Line

People react differently to the finish line. A lot of people see it and get that last push, a second or third wind, and they ramp up and cross it like a racehorse! If you're in the front of the pack, there are a lot of people gathered to cheer you on. There's energy and encouragement there. As more runners cross the line, the crowd thins out and the energy begins to fade.

Others see the finish line and wonder if they can make it. It's true. You would think running that far and being able to see it would give someone energy. If you've never run a race, it can be emotional. The longer the race, the more draining it can be. There's a level of mental toughness and grit that goes with the sport. Second guessing the finish may catch some off guard. You've seen the footage of a runner coming around that last turn and just collapsing or breaking down. The emotion wasn't anticipated and if it's your first race or early in the sport for you, there's really no way to know that you'll react that way. This is also why you will see runners who have completed the race go back to find partners, teammates, family, etc. who are participating and finish the race with them.

Some come across the finish line very quietly. The crowd is no longer there. There may or may not be someone waiting for them. By this point in the race, the end of the group is very spread out. Sometimes you don't even get to meet and make yourself a quick finish-line buddy. It's just you, finishing what you set out to do.

And then there are those who don't finish at all. Some get injured and can't. Some weren't feeling well to start with and couldn't overcome their ailment to be able to finish. Some didn't have the mental stamina to finish the race. And there are some who, for many reasons we don't know, just couldn't finish. No one starts a race intending not to finish. Read that again. **No one starts a race intending not to finish.**

Most know the real competition is with yourself. If you're a beginner, you need a base time. If you've done this for a while you are trying to beat your previous times. All the while trying to improve to get to the level of finishing or placing in your group in the race.

No one starts their weight loss journey without intending to finish. No one!

Nobody says, "I'm going to lose 25 pounds" with the intention of giving up. Nobody!

Every New Year's Resolution, New Year New You, I'm starting now, I've got to get this weight off, whatever the declaration is that's made to the world is done with every fiber of someone's being and belief.

So why doesn't this race get finished? Why do so many not reach the finish line? Why do those who do reach the finish line find themselves starting all over again instead of improving and becoming competitive?

It's because most treat it like a race. There's a start, a course, and a finish line. When we get to that finish line, we reward ourselves with all the things we were deprived of during the race, much like runners who have trained for a long time do. We party like rock stars and toss aside everything we've been doing to train and go right back to what we did to get to the starting line in the first place.

Some will stick with working out, drinking water, and some of the good habits picked up along the way. That's what yours truly did the first time. After I lost my weight, while I didn't go back to everything, I did enjoy more sweet treats and, remember, I didn't lose the soda until much later on in my health journey, not during my weight loss journey.

The "finish line" when it comes to losing weight is the most heartbreaking place for me as a coach. This is where dreams are shattered, and lives are lost. Yes, I do mean lives lost in a literal sense.

I can't tell you how many people I've watched through the years shed pounds, gain them back, shed them again, gain them back again, and eventually give up. The toll that it puts on your body is incredible. It does damage. Some of that is not reversible.

It takes a mental toll, too. I've seen too many wonderful, beautiful, capable people (men and women) succeed with their weight loss goals, gain some back, and rather than get back on track, they melt down mentally and give up. They "can't do it." They "can't keep it up." They "aren't worthy." They stop moving, depression sets in, and the slow course downhill begins.

What I'm trying to say here is this: **There is no finish line!** If you don't make permanent, lasting changes and become the person you want and need to be, you will fight this battle your entire life until you can't fight it anymore. You can get to where you don't need to study or learn much anymore. You can get to where you only need to make small adjustments to maintain your weight and lab numbers. You can get to where you don't need a coach anymore (but you stay in touch because she's crazy cool and you just bonded—it happens). What you can't do is go back to the place where food, drinks, and movement are optional and/or a free-for-all.

Tough love, from your coach.

CHAPTER 6

LEARNING THE STUFF

Now that I had a starting point, I was chomping at the bit to get going. I was doing the best I could with a sore post-op knee and a torn meniscus on the other knee. Once I got that knee going again, I discovered Zumba. It wasn't pretty, but I was moving again.

As I told you, my daughter insisted that I try this Zumba thing. I put it off for as long as I could but finally gave in. To put it nicely, it was a nightmare. I walked into that room confident that four years of cheerleading over twenty years ago would get me through this class looking like a diva. Much to my dismay, and to the further dismay of my instructor, Jessica Carillo, I looked more like a circus clown wearing a blindfold. It was awful!

I kept going to class but did not improve quickly. What was this magic that these people possessed? I know now it was years of repetition, but at the time they all seemed like the Rockettes to me. Being an overachiever and needing to at least be able to hold my own in this mystical world of dance, I took the Basic 1 license training and became an instructor. I never had any intention of teaching my own classes, I just wanted to know how to do this thing.

Turns out, knowing how to do something and actually doing it are very different. But the knowing definitely helps with the doing. It also prepared me for what was coming with my nutrition education and application. Here's what I learned:

I had to be willing to grow.

> I could not stay the same person and achieve different results. Growth is required for change.

I had to be willing to be bad at things.

> I won't say that no one is a natural at something, but very, very few can accomplish their craft, their dream, or their expertise without years of work.

This was going to take time.

> I didn't get into the position that I was in overnight, and I wasn't coming out of it overnight either.

I had to be willing to make mistakes and, more importantly, I had to be willing to learn from them.

Now, I'd had some success up to this point and you'd think that I would know those things. When you're talking about your health, your heart, your hormones, your ability to move and think straight rather than your looks, your size, do these jeans make my butt look big, this becomes a completely different ball game. This wasn't rocking a size 8 pair of jeans, gang, this was saving my life. Going in, this was intellectual. I've always been good at school and learning so I thought I'd just go out there and figure it out. In fact, I thought I'd just tweak what I'd done before and everything would be fine. But that's not how it works. Thus, the book you're reading today.

At the time I wasn't so grateful for learning these lessons through Zumba. Later on, and to this day, I am eternally grateful for them.

Zumba was set in motion—over the next few years I would go on to get my Gold, Kids, Kids, Jr., and Toning licenses. I do mix the Gold and the Toning in with my classes now. The Kids, Jr. will start for me on my grandbaby's 4th birthday. If you're wondering, the next one will be Aqua Zumba. I also have a license in Circl Mobility—stay tuned, that's coming.

About this time in my life, I ran across my mentor, Darren Hardy. I have been doing daily leadership training with him for years now and am very grateful for what I've learned there. If you are a leader in any capacity (home, church, work, community—here's a secret, we're ALL leaders), this is definitely something to check out. You can find this gold at Darren Daily, Daily Mentoring with Darren Hardy, at dd.darrenhardy.com.

Darren also has lots of training opportunities and I will tell you, I've never taken a course of his and not taken away huge, life-changing information. Put this into practice and you'll be well on your way to the kind of life you want to live.

One training in particular, Insane Productivity, is what really helped prepare me for my studies to become a nutrition coach. I'm telling you this because whatever you're trying to accomplish in your life, whether it's education, transformation, building a business, or succeeding in the field that you're already in, when you try to do more than one of these things at a time, you need some crazy good skills. Insane Productivity delivers on that. Those were skills that I not only needed then, but have continued to use since.

Now I've got some study skills, I started gathering information, starting with the book from Mom's office. Looking back now, the journey was rather interesting. At times it looked like I had squirreled off onto other paths, but it all came together nicely. Even better, as my journey continues, the information keeps coming in right on time, just when I need it.

Working my way through this, I knew in my heart that I was going to figure this out for myself. By "figure this out for myself," I mean that I knew the Lord would guide me and that He'd already given me the ability to think, reason, and know when I was on the right track. Being blessed with the knowledge and ability to turn my situation around, I would use this to help others. I don't know about you, but it upsets me to bury people who had a lot more to give to this world but couldn't figure out how to get their health back. I also know that there are some, no matter how dire the situation, who won't listen or care about what I have to say. It's unfortunate, but it's also OK. We must walk our own paths and our own journeys. I'm telling you now, this girl wants to go out like she's stealing home plate!

Beginning with the book *How to Heal Cancer with Nutrition* by Patrick Quillin, I began, slowly, to transform my life. It was a tough read for me, and I'll be honest, I've yet to finish it. I don't read books like most people, especially when I'm searching for specific information. Let's just say when I'm on a mission there are 3"x5" cards, sections highlighted, pages marked for reference, and each reference followed up on specifically. I will read the book in its entirety someday but that's going to involve a beach and unlimited time. Maybe now that I have some years and miles it won't be so difficult for me to read. Regardless, it started the journey.

As I mentioned before, through this book I was introduced to Dr. Tom O'Bryan. He's a great guy and you should look him up. Lots of great information about the toxins of our world, how they affect us, and how we can protect ourselves. A fun fact about me is that my water bottle is glass. A lot of people ask about that, wonder if I worry about breaking it (I've lost three of these so far), and just don't get why I would go to the trouble. Well, I was already anti-plastic before I read the book *You Can Fix Your Brain*, but now I really am. About the only time you'll see me with plastic water bottles is when I travel. Although, if I put my glass one in my checked bag, I can at least enjoy it at my destination. Lots of good information in this book, on his website, and in his trainings on the blood-brain barrier, toxins, and our overall health.

Dr. O'Bryan was promoting a health summit not long after I purchased his book. If you've never participated in one, I recommend that you do. Keep in mind, there are a lot of them out there and you can spend a lot of time going through these so pick and choose wisely or you'll become overwhelmed. If the topic specifically interests you (for me that was diabetes, heart disease, and nutrition) then invest in the package where you can have access to it forever. Yes, at some point you won't go back to it anymore, but there's a lot of information there and it's worth getting so that you can go through it thoroughly and apply what you need to your life. You can also just reach out to a coach, like me, who will share information with you because she wants to see you healthy and thriving. At the summit, I signed up and watched the *iThrive!* docuseries and it changed my life. It's also the reason I was able to reverse my pre-diabetic diagnosis before my next round of labs. That's less than six months folks!

iThrive!, I believe, is where I became connected with Dr. Joel Fuhrman. Dr. Fuhrman has treated many patients with diabetes and heart disease with excellent results. He promotes whole food, plant-based eating and the science behind it is crazy cool, as are the results. I spent about 60 to 90 days eating this way and it's life-changing, gang, it really is. I also knew that, being from Oklahoma, my husband had three smokers on the deck and the likelihood that I would be meat-free for life was slim. But I don't eat nearly as much meat as I used to, and my health says it all. Eat those plants people, it's where the magic happens!

Now that my journey had taken me this far, I was hungry (no pun intended). I wanted the truth, I wanted to be healthy, and I wanted to do that with food. Before I found myself with a less-than-desirable diagnosis, I did not trust standard medicine. After what I had learned up to this point, I really didn't. Don't get me wrong, with my background in workers' compensation injuries I know many great orthopedic doctors and if a bone is protruding from my body, I'm making that call. But when it comes to sniffles, allergies, even a sinus infection, I'm going to rely on my body which was wonderfully made to do what it knows it needs to do to heal. I'm also going to give it what it needs in order to do that. If something continues, then yes, I will see a doctor and, if necessary, I will take a prescription medication. What I won't do is walk into a room with a doctor who picks up their script pad while I'm talking. They can take notes, or they can listen, but when that pad comes out we're done. I've walked out of appointments because of it. Doctors work for you; remember that.

I've been very fortunate to have found my doctor, who not only works with me on this journey but will let me talk about my learning and direct me to where I can learn further if I want to. Find a doctor like that, they're out there!

Once my passion was ignited, and I had found natural remedies that work, I then learned about Precision Nutrition. Once again, it was perfectly timed with my journey and this is where I got my nutrition coaching certification. I spent a lot of time comparing different programs and this one just spoke to me. I can utilize their methods with someone who just wants to lose some fluff prior to an occasion, someone who wants to get serious about their health, or someone who wants to sculpt a body to compete with. I really enjoyed the program and dove right in. It took me just over a year to get that coaching certification. Remember, I was working a full-time job at the time. My studies and testing usually took place during my lunch break. What's your lunch hour doing for you?

I don't think I've been so proud to have a certificate in my life! And although I wanted to run out and be coach to the world, I had work to do for myself. Just like the flight attendant tells you to put your oxygen mask on first, you can't help someone else until you have done what it takes to help yourself stay alive first. Although I had made great strides, I knew that I wouldn't wait for perfection, but I needed to make sure I was settled because adding the coaching to my already busy life was going to add stress. Yeah, remember that? What do you know? The girl can be taught.

Before we move on, I want to add something here. My three core values are growth, health, and impact. Prior to these events, I hadn't grown much. In a way, finding out some bad news about my health helped me turn around not only physically, but mentally and spiritually as well. If you aren't living in alignment with your core values you're living in conflict. Let that sink in.

CHAPTER 7

DOING THE STUFF

Knowledge is not power.
Knowledge + action = power

While learning all the things I needed to do to reverse my diagnosis and regain my health, I found myself in a happy spot. I love learning and growing, and it felt good to be back in that practice. However, I knew that if I didn't take action on what I had learned, I'd be in the same boat as before and eventually cruise off into the sunset for good. And much earlier than I'd like set sail.

Some of you may be wondering how long it took me to learn this stuff. I'd love to be able to answer that for you. But I can't. This is an ongoing process. No, I don't study for hours like I used to, and yes, I found what would work for me and for my body. Keep in mind that science is constantly moving forward, and new things are always emerging. No, I don't live in a state of FOMO, but I do keep an eye on things. As we age, our bodies and metabolisms change, and it doesn't hurt to keep a growth mindset when it comes to what will serve our body and our health. So yes,

I'm still learning, but I do know enough that I can help others navigate their personal chemistry and get results for weight loss, lowering blood sugar, and starting to move again. I will forever be a student of this.

I've mentioned before that I'm an overachiever and a perfectionist. Not always the best combo. However, I knew that in order to make progress I had to start, take a step, and try some things. I knew I would learn along the way, and I knew that it didn't have to be perfect, it just had to be started.

If you're reading this and waiting for that perfect start date (New Years, birthday, a month before a high school reunion, a wedding, etc.), I would strongly recommend right now that you STOP!

Stop waiting
Stop looking for that magic pill
Stop trying to learn it all before you even try
Stop trying to out-exercise a crappy diet
Stop making excuses

Just start already…seriously. Even if you only do one healthy (or healthier) thing today and that's the only thing you do until it becomes a habit, and you pick another thing and work on that until it's a habit, you have set in motion things that will benefit you. Maybe you can handle a few things at once. The point is:

Start
Start today
Start with one thing
Stay with that one thing until it's part of your life

Just start already.

Let me be completely honest with you here. Your mindset—getting your head in the game—is the most critical part of getting your health back. Yes, being scared of a diagnosis will motivate you. It'll get you moving, thinking, and looking for answers, but it will not *keep* you moving in the right direction. I had to get real in my head. I had to give myself permission. This was going to take time, effort, investment (of finances as well as time), and I had to know why. Why was I going to do this? Why did I want to live longer? Why did I not want to have to deal with diabetes? What was the purpose of getting my heart health under control?

The first thing I did was to find my why.

I want to go to out either used up (like the little old lady that goes to sleep and crosses over) or serving full force and taken out. I want my life to mean something. When someone is standing there talking at my memorial, I don't want them to have to search for things to say. I want it said that I cared, I loved, I served, and I reached as many people as I could so that they could live full lives. I want it said that I was there for my kids, my grandkids, and, Lord willing, my great-grandkids (and hey, five generations isn't uncommon on one side of my family, so yes, I would be so blessed to know my great- great-grandchildren). I want to play with the younger generations. I want to guide and direct those below me as they age. I want to share the joy of dance, movement, and health until I just can't anymore. I want to give life back to those who thought that they had lost it. By life, I mean quality of life. We don't know when we're going to die, but I want to go out like I'm trying to steal home plate. I want to leave a legacy of a life lived fully; to give inspiration to others, and for them to have memories of me being there and able to interact fully, both physically and mentally. I want helping others to be able to be my full-time work. I'd like to make enough money to fund a foundation to help those who can't afford coaching so that they can change their legacy. This all lines up with my core values of growth, impact, and health. Finding my why was the most critical of "doing the things."

What's your why? Looking hot is not wrong, but it's not going to carry you through the long haul.

The second thing I did was return to what I knew.

In my 30s I lost eight dress sizes. I literally became half the person, size-wise, that I had been. So, that was my base for getting started. I know now that I could have done it better and in a healthier way. But much of what I did then became part of my life, so I knew that returning to that baseline would at least move me in the right direction. One thing I'm proud to say that I never, ever quit doing is drinking water. I'm not sure why I picked a gallon a day—not telling you that's the right or perfect amount (we're all different)—but that has been consistent for me since the beginning. So I gave myself a gold star for that and was happy that I wasn't starting from scratch. I also knew how to create a calorie deficit and I did that again. Getting the weight off would help with a few issues and I knew I'd find my way on the rest of them. Some of the health resolutions took longer than others. But I had to start somewhere, and this wasn't a bad place to start.

The third thing I did was to learn.

We covered that earlier, so I'll move on. Again, keep in mind, a growth mindset is an asset here. Our bodies change, science and medicine change—learn to keep learning and growing.

The fourth thing I did was to do.

Everyone's body is different. What works for one may not work for another. There are a LOT of puzzle pieces here. So, as I would learn, I would apply. If it worked, great. If it didn't, I let that be OK.

I mentioned before that I did a whole food, plant-based diet for 30 days. It was a game changer. It greatly improved my health. I still eat using that method to this day. But I do like meat, and I wanted to figure out how to keep it in my life. So I've played with that over the years and have found a good balance with it at this time. At least my lab work and body seem to agree.

Currently I try to keep my breakfast 50% protein and 50% fruits or vegetables. This is visual, not actual macros. Lunch is similar, allowing for some healthy fats. Dinner is similar to breakfast. Do I get this accurate every time? No, I don't. Do I snack? Sometimes, yes, I do. But I know how to choose my food outside of this regimen so that it doesn't spike my blood sugar. When you keep that spike from happening, it serves not only your blood sugar levels but also your fat-burning ability. No more midafternoon slumps and plenty of energy for my day (including workouts), and inflammation and joint pain are things of the past.

Exercise became consistent in my life. Not just for losing weight, but the movement helped my joints and my stamina. Since running was no longer a smart option for my knee (seriously, try running with a screw in your leg, it's not comfortable—for those of you who can, I'm supportively jealous), and the treadmill is not only boring but painful as well, I started dancing. If someone had told me I'd be into dance fitness and someday instructing a class of my own, I would have laughed. But fortunately, my daughter did not give up on me and my group is fun, sweet, and thriving. Zumba gave me my knee back. It let me move again. It let me connect with wonderful people and keeps a smile on my face.

As much as I love Zumba, cardio is not enough. Yes, we work muscle groups and focus on fitness-oriented routines in class. Bone and muscle health are important and resistance training is a must. It also affects the scale, but the trade-off is worth it. As of the writing of this book I am back on the weight bench, utilizing resistance bands, doing bodyweight workouts and focusing on my muscle. It took years to get back the ability to build muscle. Yes folks, my hormones were shot to the point that building muscle was next to impossible. I'm grateful to have that back and now have added it back into my routine. I won't kid you here, this is lifelong. Here and there won't get it done.

Part of the fun is that I've tried so many types of workouts. Continuing to change things up really helps your body and your mind. Don't worry about being bad at something. Just do it and keep doing it until you get it. Your bones and your body will appreciate you for that. Plus, you won't get bored, so that's a bonus.

Another thing I did was to eliminate soda. THIS…WAS…HARD! It took many tries, lots of grace, and I highly recommend

Excedrin Migraine Relief tablets. If you have been drinking soda for many years, it takes some doing to just set it to the side. For my diet soda friends out there, lose it. Yes, you are eliminating the sugar. However, the brain doesn't know the difference between artificial sweetener and sugar, so you still crave carbs and sweets. This book isn't about the dangers of soda, but look it up some time. There is zero nutritional value or benefit to this stuff at all.

Stress was something I had to get under control. Stress contributes to the following:

- Insomia – rest is critical folks
- Body soreness – "uptight" is a word for a reason
- Rapid heartbeat – that ticker should go fast when you work it, not when you're sitting still
- Depression – something I've dealt with as an adult (I now know why)
- Obesity – when you're stressed, you crave comfort food
- High blood pressure – goes along with that heart thing
- Fatigue – when your brain never shuts off, it wears you out completely

There's more, but that's plenty. This is another ongoing process in my life. I'm a people pleaser, so some of the stress I've created for myself. I don't want to let people down and I say yes to way too many things. I've worked hard to get some balance back and will continue to work on that. What I will tell you here is this: When and where you can eliminate stress or simplify your life, DO IT! Cortisol and adrenaline are hormones that we need; they serve a purpose, and that's to keep us alive. Unfortunately, just like the brain doesn't know the difference between sugar and artificial sweetener, it doesn't know the difference between good stress and bad stress. Keep it simple and your health and weight will respond kindly. Life brings enough stress, both good and bad; let's not add to it.

The three R's is another avenue I've gone down. Rest, recovery, and relaxation are things I've not valued properly in the past. I'm not talking about binging Netflix for an entire weekend (not that there's anything wrong with that), but when exercise is part of your daily life and you are constantly mindful of your health, you've got to unplug sometimes. These three R's will refresh your mind and restore your body.

These are some of the many things that I've done to get my health back and lose the weight that needed to come off. Let me get real with you right here and now—I did not wake up on January 1st one year and tackle all of this at once. To lose weight permanently you have to make life changes. Anyone can create a calorie deficit and lose some pounds. The reason people drop some weight and then gain it (and more) back is because the changes they made are not sustainable. Yes, it takes more time to lose weight this way. But if it doesn't come back, isn't it worth it?

I work on one or two things at a time until they are part of my life. I'm successful with most, but some I have to set aside and try again later. That's OK! If dropping 20 pounds would be life-saving and life changing, then work on that and get that done first. Using nutrition for that will help you in the long run with the rest of what you need to do. Once you get one thing down, move on to the next. I like to set three to four health goals a year, preferably ones that build on each other. Once I get one down, I'm ready to step up to the next level. Health goals include nutrition, exercise, rest and recovery, relaxation, training, and learning.

Where I am at today took years of dedication and determination. It's simple, but it's not easy. I will tell you though, it's absolutely worth it.

CHAPTER 8

PROGRESS, NOT PERFECTION

"Without continual growth and progress, such words as improvement, achievement, and success have no meaning."
—Benjamin Franklin

We all want to reach our goals quickly. If I could tell you how to drop 20 pounds quickly, keep it off, and get six-pack abs at the same time, believe me, this would be a great, short book, because I would gladly share that. That doesn't exist and we know it.

Some of you will read this book, get your act together, lose the weight, and keep it off because you made life changes. Others will do well for a while and then go back to their comfort zone and regain the weight. Still others will be motivated but lost and may or may not make the changes they need to for a better life. Last but not least, some will read this, put the book down, and do nothing. Each of these options is a journey.

Listen, you didn't get to be overweight or struggling with your health overnight. Where you are at now took years and many decisions. I'll give some of you the benefit of not knowing better due to circumstances growing up. But at some point in your life (aka adulthood) you're in the driver's seat, you make the calls, and you reap the consequences. I've heard it said, "You get to make the choices, but you don't get to choose the consequences." I'm not sure who penned that but it's right on the mark. But oh, the fun we had getting to this point! Let's be honest here—chips, cookies, cake, soda, all the ooey, gooey, sugary things are fun to eat! Should you never enjoy any of these things again? No, in fact, you should enjoy things that bring you pleasure. However, these are not daily items and certainly not two-out-of-three-meals a-day items. And…you know that.

"Life is a journey, not a destination."

My first weight loss journey was just that—it was strictly about weight loss. I thought I knew the things and turns out, yes, I knew how to lose weight. But I didn't know how to lose it and maintain my health. Keep in mind, I never regained all the weight back. I did get to a point in my life where my body changed (again— ladies, am I right?) and just having a calorie deficit wasn't enough. Technically, I was malnourished, and my body paid the price.

My second journey was a health journey. Yes, I needed to lose weight. But I needed nourishment more than I needed to lose weight. So, a beautiful, enlightening, and quite fulfilling journey began for me. This journey released me from the need to be perfect. That couldn't happen. The puzzle pieces weren't all in place, so I had to be OK with this path being more like a cha cha than a choreographed line dance. Some days it was sloppy, other days went so well an Olympic coach would have been proud. Each day presented new choices, more to learn, options to seek, and growth.

Let's go back to The Compound Effect and see progress in motion: *"It's not the big things that add up in the end; it's the hundreds, thousands, or millions of little things that separate the ordinary from the extraordinary."* —Darren Hardy

You're not ready to completely overhaul your diet, which, by the way, you shouldn't do all at once anyway. So, you make a commitment to eliminate 100 calories a day from your diet. You're a predictable creature and eat pretty much similar things on similar days, and you've been tracking so you know where you can cut 100 calories. Just 100 calories, we're not talking something drastic here. That's skipping the cheese on a burger, not having chips at the Mexican restaurant (wait, what?!?), eating an apple instead of a piece of cheesecake. You get the idea. If you cut just 100 calories from your daily diet, you'll lose roughly 10 pounds in a year without much effort (or tears) at all. Add a 15-minute walk daily to burn another 100 calories and we're talking 20 pounds. Two changes, two choices, twenty pounds gone! Inertia has been broken! Hey folks, that's the hardest part, so if you're there, no matter how frustrated you get, keep going. Because going back to sitting still will take that and more effort to restart. You can do this!

Now we're cooking! When you start to notice, or even better when others start to notice, you have momentum. Momentum is a beautiful thing. It means that you've started movement and now can continue moving on your own. Did you know that it takes more fuel to launch the space shuttle than it does for it to fly its entire mission? It takes tons of steam to get a train moving but once it's moving it takes very little to keep going. We are much the same. Once that movement is in motion, you start seeing some cool things like the notch going up on your belt, loose jeans, shoulder seams on your shirts have moved, you know, the cool stuff; now you start to make other choices to do more. You start:

- Adding more protein to your meals.
- Swapping chips with cut up veggies.
- Hummus takes the place of ranch (yes, I realize that is borderline blasphemy to some of my readers, I promise you'll live).
- Pizza ordered as a medium rather than a large.

The list goes on. There are literally hundreds of choices you can make to improve your nutrition or reduce calories daily.

And then, it happens—insert record scratch sound here—the boss sends you on a trip for work or it's time for the family vacay or there's a wedding, funeral, or family reunion. Your head starts spinning, your heart rate goes up, you know that you are about to be totally surrounded by food or have to navigate others providing food or eating in restaurants for days. This is where progress over perfection comes in.

You've built some skills. You've been making the choices. Regardless of your circumstances you can use them anywhere. Maybe you don't feel comfortable? You don't want to draw attention to yourself. You don't want to hurt your mother's, aunt's, cousin's, or whoever's feelings by not eating their special casserole or sheet cake. You know what I'm talking about here. Or it's the holidays. It starts on Halloween with the invasion of tiny candy, and it goes until New Year's Eve.

You have a choice here, friends. Do the best you can, use smaller plates, learn some skills around what order to eat your food in or how to pair it (something I specialize in) or, for the duration of the event or occasion, eat the food, connect with family, friends, or colleagues, and enjoy the meal. Let's say it's dinner. So have a stellar breakfast and lunch and go enjoy. Start back with that stellar breakfast the next day and continue with your meals as you normally do. Maybe it's lunch brought in at the office. Breakfast rocks and dinner is light and healthy. Didn't get a walk in today? No worries, walk further or for a longer time tomorrow. Or walk the same, just don't skip a week, a month or a year just because you missed a day.

Whether you're changing your nutrition for weight loss or health purposes, the odds of having 365 perfect days year after year is not reasonable. The expectation is too high. Some extra calories here and there will not undo everything you've accomplished unless you quit completely and stay in that mode. Yes, a nutrition coach told you to enjoy a family or holiday meal, guilt free. This coach is also telling you to get back on track the next meal or at the very latest the next day. Do not, absolutely do not, deprive yourself. Do value yourself and get back to where you were as quickly as possible.

Fitness works the same way. If you've been on the couch for a year or more, you're not going to go out and walk a 5K. You might, but it will hurt. But you can start walking for five or ten minutes. You can start parking at the end of the parking lot and walking up to the store, around it, and back to the car. Even if you can't do these things daily, if you do them as often as you can, you will start to see progress. Now you can up your time or start measuring your distance. Keep going, keep adding, keep progressing.

Weights, start small. Maybe you don't even have weights. A half-gallon milk jug filled with water is four pounds. It makes a great kettlebell. Start with 30-day challenges with short sets of exercise and then work up from there. My Zumba students are told to modify and not worry about the arms when they start. If they need to rest, they do it. I can't tell you how many have started my classes and not been able to do a full class at the beginning. Now they're the ones encouraging the new students and letting them know it's OK to take a break while they are finishing the class. Some of them are out-dancing *me* now!

We start where we are.

People are going to offer you advice. Listen, look it up for yourself, make informed decisions. Someone may mention something, and you try it. Maybe it works, maybe it doesn't. You haven't lost anything by trying something new. Remember that I was learning and doing along the way and changed my practices as I went. There's not a one size fits all. People mean well, but as humans we don't always remember that there is not a cookie cutter scenario here. One method will work for some, while other methods work for others. You gotta do you here. Don't argue. Don't try to persuade someone to your way of doing things. While your genes don't determine your destiny, they do determine how your body will respond to nutrition and fitness.

Look into what this well-meaning person has to say, see if you can use some, all, or none of it, be gracious about it, and do you.

If you have a cold or a fever, you shouldn't work out at all, and I certainly wouldn't be overly worried about food. Eat what you can and will eat. Get back on track later. If you can move, great, do it. If you can't, don't worry about it.

When we stress about not doing things perfectly, when we get worked up about missing a workout or eating in a way that isn't the healthiest or in line with what we're trying to accomplish, we add to the problem. Remember our friend cortisol. It's a great tool but it doesn't know that we're stressing because we're trying to be better. It just knows that we're stressing and goes to work. Don't sweat things that are out of your control or the small things that you can catch up on later.

Progress over perfection.

> *"Perfection is the enemy of progress."*
> —Winston Churchill

CHAPTER 9

THE BEAUTY OF CHANGE

"The beauty of change is found in the metamorphosis. You have to start as a caterpillar before you can become a butterfly."
—Unknown

Change—a single word that can send shivers down our spine in an instant. We are creatures of habit. We are creatures of comfort. We will fight change, even if it's for our good, with every fiber of our being. Our bodies don't like change. The human body wants to stay on autopilot. It's a survival thing hardwired in us from the dawn of time.

In the past, people's lives were very consistent from beginning to end. Location, beliefs, customs, and traditions passed down from generation to generation worked and there just wasn't much need to change. A great invention would come along now and then, and if it was one that affected home life, it was welcomed with open arms. We can handle one change at a time if we have enough time to embrace it and get used to it. Nowadays, computers are in need of an upgrade every one to one and a half years and speed of production is picking up. You can buy a television one year and go back to the store the following year and there's a whole new crop that will do all kinds of new things. How fast are our cell phones changing? It's hard to keep up, right? It took much longer for us to go from the flip phone to the Razr than it does now to go from smart phones to phones that will do more and more. Technology, diversity, economy, politics, society, how we work and learn, all of these things are changing and they're doing it fast. It's enough to make your head spin.

So, while we're keeping up with all of that, we decide to make some personal changes. Life changes, health changes, fitness changes, you name it. That's a lot of change going on. Some change is out of our control. Some must happen in order for us to be able to keep up to support our families. It's no wonder that making changes for a healthier you gets pushed to the back burner or it's attempted over and over and it's the one thing you allow yourself to give up on. But let's be fair here, if you don't do something about your health, change is going to happen anyway. You can live with prescriptions for a while to help you out, but at some point, not eating right and not moving your body is going to cause you to be sick. You'll miss work, you might lose a digit or a limb, your eyesight can be at risk, you may end up in a wheelchair. Are those the kinds of changes you want to work with?

You didn't get to the point of needing to work on your health overnight. It took years. It took decisions. Part of it was just life itself. For example, when you were a kid, how much did you play outside? What's crazy is that the chick writing this book used to play outside all day, everyday when school wasn't going on. Younger generations will have a much different answer. The point is, when we were young, we moved much more. Then high school hits. If we're not doing sports, we slow down even more. Then we graduate. Ever hear of the freshman 15? Yeah, it's a thing for a reason. Fast food, stress from studies, being completely uprooted from family and friends, and fatigue factor in here. Maybe you didn't do college, so the next step would be adulting. The fulltime job (the majority of which now are sedentary), getting your own place, finding someone to spend your life with, all the things.

All of those things cause change. It's necessary and it seems subtle. It was what it was. Let's say you've got the job or career, the spouse, the house, the car, and now you're thinking about kids. How many young couples do you know of who sat down and talked about how they're going to eat? I don't know of any. No, you merge what each of you ate growing up, try things from each side, decide what works for you, and that's what ends up on the table. For some, that's after you even learn how to cook those things. For those of you out there, and I see this more and more now, that do talk about food and what goes on the table when you cross the kiddo threshold, kudos to you! Obesity is becoming a real problem for children and our younger generation seems to have an eye on that. Thank you for that and I promise to be that extended grandma or aunt that tries to work with it and not sugar your kid up before you pick them up.

Now the kiddos are in grade school, all the fun things are going on, your belly is growing, you're on your fourth set of bigger clothes, you can hardly keep up with the kids, your job, the house, the yard, and the new pup. Some, at this point, are even looking at divorce. Because, let's face it, you've changed. You go to the doctor, he or she recommends dropping some weight (again), and you leave with shiny new scripts for blood pressure and cholesterol meds. What the heck happened?

I realize this might have happened on a different timeline for some, but you get the idea. I also realize some did not marry or have children. The point is, a lot of life happens; changes get made while living life and you don't even realize it

So, let's be fair about this change thing. Not all change is painful. In fact, some of the changes I've talked about were quite fun. The changes you need to make now are forced. They are associated with turning a negative back into a positive. So, we're already on the wrong foot with the wrong mindset here.

Now, you're a smart person and the doc made some recommendations about what to do, so you start with that. I mean this respectfully: Many doctors have very little training in nutrition. They went to school to learn medicine, not nutrition. There are just not many hours required for nutrition training in pre-med or med school. What they instructed you to do was meant with all of the best intentions and they believe it was good advice. Here's the problem—they're not planning on seeing you again for another year, they've given you the same instructions they've given a hundred other patients, and they didn't get a background on your lifestyle. Some will refer you to a nutrition coach, nutritionist, or maybe even a dietitian. What I'm getting at here is you need to change not only your fitness level but your food as well. You cannot out-exercise a bad diet. You might be thin, but thin does not equal healthy.

Doctors are respected members of our community. Go back to

our tribal wiring, and you'll find them higher up in the tribe. Your doctor studied a LOT, and they are smart. They are also human, have time constraints on how much time they can spend with you, and they are your hired medical advisor. In other words, they work for you. Go into your appointments with questions written down. Don't rely on your memory or you'll get lost in conversation and forget to ask. Use your patient portal. Find a doctor who will help you find the answers if they don't know them. It took me a long time to find a doctor who could truly help me with my health issues. Take your time, find a good one, become a team.

This is where change gets beautiful.

Let's start out with a shift in mindset. You don't *have* to work out, you don't *have* to change the way you eat—you *get* to. You have discovered early enough that you can do something about your health, and now you have the opportunity to be the best version of yourself. Yep, you had some fun getting here, and let me tell you that you can still have fun. You're just going to do it a little differently going forward.

Here are some misconceptions about changing your health, along with some new ways of thinking about them.

Eating healthy doesn't taste good.

Eating healthy gives me the opportunity to explore new foods, new recipes, and different ways of making my favorite recipes to nourish my body.

Have you ever heard of herbs and spices? Yeah, they add great flavor to your food, and they have amazing health benefits. Unless a recipe calls for salt and it's an active part of the ingredients, only salt your food when you eat it. The salt will be on top, you get the satisfaction of the flavor, and you reduce your intake significantly. Cooking with spices and herbs takes some learning, but it's so worth it. Here are a few that will help you with your health goals and keep your food tasty:

Black Peppercorn	Adds a kick and may reduce cancer risk
Cayenne Pepper	Helps maintain healthy weight and improves heart health
Cinnamon	Reduces added sugars, helps control blood sugar and blood pressure
Cloves	Reduces arthritis risk, decreases oxidative stress, supports eye health
Coriander	May help protect against cognitive decline, cancer, and mood disorders
Garlic	Lowers high blood pressure, supports immunity
Ginger	May help soothe nausea, fight arthritis pain, sooth migraines
Oregano	Reduces inflammation, helps fight infections
Paprika	May help decrease inflammation and pain

Peppermint	Helps boost mood, improve focus, relieve IBS symptoms, and ease nausea
Rosemary	Helps brain function and mood
Turmeric	Helps ease inflammation and lower type 2 diabetes risk

I don't like vegetables and five servings of fruits and vegetables doesn't leave room for much else.

This is my time to learn how to prepare vegetables in a way that I will enjoy. I get to incorporate fruits and vegetables in my diet to benefit from the power of plants and let them heal my body.

Remember when your mom and maybe your grandma told you to eat your vegetables? She wasn't kidding. Plant foods are powerful! They are cost-effective, help to lower body mass index, blood pressure, and cholesterol, and keep your blood sugar in check. Not to mention the vitamins and antioxidants that are packed into fruits and vegetables. Now, I know some of you are concerned about fruit having natural sugar. But fruit also has fiber which slows the sugar intake down. Knowing when to eat fruit and what to pair it with will help even more with that. So, if you find that fruit causes you to spike, try eating it at the end of a meal or pairing it with healthy fats such as nut butters. It's a game-changer.

Here are some ways to get more of these great foods into your diet.

Eat more stir fry!

Use them in soups, pasta sauces, and casseroles.

Add to whole grain muffins or pancakes.

Veggies can be used in place of pasta. There's a bit of a learning curve here, but it's worth it. I make lasagna now with zucchini rather than pasta. It's delicious, has no texture difference, and is so much better for you.

Veggies can also be added to smoothies. While the color takes some getting used to, you can't taste them.

I just don't have time to work out.

Time is the most precious commodity there is aside from health. I accept the challenge to find time to move my body during the day even if it's only for five to ten minutes at a time. I also accept the challenge to take a look at my life and see if priorities can be rearranged to allow more time for self-care.

You will lose this argument with me every single time. When I lost eight dress sizes, I was a single mom, with two very active, very school- and church-involved pre-teens. I said the same thing. I was tired of being fat, tired of not liking who and what I saw in the mirror, and tired of being tired. I remember specifically asking God to just show me what I need to do to lose some weight. He delivered. I was sitting at Super Cuts waiting on my turn and picked up a copy of *Shape Magazine*. Wouldn't you know, there it was in black and white. There was more to the article but what stuck in my head was that I needed to walk for 45 to 60 minutes for a minimum of five days a week. I gave proper thanks, got my hair cut, and my wheels started spinning. Where in the world was I going to find 45 minutes to move? Back then there wasn't Fitbit, and we hadn't really grasped the fact that the time frame could be cut into sections. Some talked about it, but it wasn't really a thing yet.

I was too broke for new shoes or workout clothes or fancy gadgets. Plus, I had vowed I would not buy a size bigger, so I worked with what I had. I started walking. That's it, I just walked. When you're not used to doing much of anything, that first week of five 45-minute walks is tough. Today, I don't recommend it, but I was on a mission, young, and didn't have much fitness training, so that's what I did. I had lifted weights and played sports in high school and was also following some of the ladies in the fitness world at that time. Denise Austin and Rachel McLish will forever hold a special place in my heart. Ladies, thank you. I just didn't have the formal training. *Shape* said to walk, so I walked.

I walked after work on the days the kids were at home. They were old enough to be at home alone for that long and I walked around the block so that I could be close. We still had a landline phone and the only cell phone we had went with me on the walk. On pretty days when school or homework wasn't a factor, I walked at a park around the playground so I could keep an eye on them. On practice days I walked around the field. In the winter I walked around the basketball court, in the hall, or on the bleachers. When it rained, I walked in the house. If I was fortunate enough for them to have an activity, I could get to the gym to use the treadmill if the weather was bad, and if time would allow. I walked at work during lunch. I even walked the stairs. In the beginning, I'd have to walk in place on the landing before I could go up again. I walked and walked and walked. Eventually, the weight started coming off. I added weights to my efforts. I lifted during TV shows, while dinner was cooking, wherever I could find 15 to 20 minutes to pick up a dumbbell or do some bodyweight exercises.

Nowadays, we know that the time can be split up. Yes, 45 minutes worth of cardio is excellent, but if you don't have it, you don't have it. Something always, always, always trumps nothing! ALWAYS!

You don't have to do 45 minutes five days a week. At least not when starting out. I tell my clients and my dance fitness students all the time, you start where you are. This is oversimplified, but here's what you do:

Find some time, any time.

Move, lift, use resistance bands, stretch, dance, something.

Find something that you like, you'll stick with it longer.

Here are some ways to sneak exercise into your day. This is not an all-inclusive list. Be creative, have fun, and just find ways to move.

Take the stairs	Have walking meetings
Walk when you're on the phone	Clean the house
Park far away	Stretch at your desk
Lift at your desk	Lift while watching TV

More ideas to help you get moving:

Make it a game.

Come up with goals for your day or create a group and challenge each other.

Do a step challenge with a group.

Fitbit does not do challenges anymore, but you can set one up on Stridekick for your friends with fitness trackers. It works with any brand of tracker.

Sign up for a fitness class.

If you pay for it, you're more likely to do it. Grab a buddy and make it fun.

Get up early.

Waking up an hour earlier will allow you time to work out before anyone (including yourself) knows what you're doing.

It's too expensive.

It's fortunate that improving one's health with food and exercise doesn't have to cost any money to start.

Yep, that's right. You can start right here, right now, with ZERO money. Use what you have, buy different groceries, and get going.

I started with a decent pair of tennis shoes and wore them completely out. To celebrate hitting the 10-pounds-lost mark, I bought myself a new pair of tennis shoes. I wore sweats or shorts that I already had. Shirts and jackets, same thing. You do not need to go buy an entire Under Armour, Adidas, or Nike wardrobe to work out in. You don't have to go buy equipment. You don't have to have a gym membership. You don't even need to buy bottled water. On this note, however, I would prefer you have some sort of filtration system to make sure your water is clean. But it's not necessary to start.

"Eating healthy is more expensive" is a myth. The reason it seems more expensive is that you likely don't have everything you need for that healthy recipe in the beginning, so initially you have to buy more. When you switch over to eating better your food needs change. You start to buy the things that you know you're going to make. Eventually, your kitchen pantry and refrigerator make the shift and you have what you need on hand more often.

When you get your health back in line you start to save money in other areas.

You don't have to buy new sizes of clothes all the time. You'll balance out and can buy nice things that last longer because you're not wearing clothes out or changing sizes.

You won't spend as much time or money at the doctor. Twice a year is usually all the time I spend with my doctor. In the beginning it might be more due to monitoring, but once you've figured things out, you'll be distant friends with your doc rather than feeling like shoe-shopping buddies.

Prescription expenses go down because you won't need as much or as many, and you could possibly eliminate that expense altogether.

Cooking at home eliminates expensive eating out. At this point in time, a salad costs as much as a burger. It's expensive to eat out. I challenge you to make a salad that costs $14.99 for the entire salad that you can enjoy for several meals. Now you can save money by cooking at home and go out to someplace nice for celebrations and occasions.

If you really want to take your game to the next level, grow some of your own food. Seeds are cheap and fresh food is amazing. So are fresh herbs and spices, which can be grown inside. Plants are cheap and they give back with oxygen and by being used in your food. Enjoy!

I don't know what to do or where to start.

The book in my hands is enough to get me headed in the right direction. I'm fortunate to live in a time in which, with the correct online or social media search, I can connect with those who have gone before me, lost weight naturally, and improved their health.

It's not *that* you Google, it's *what* you Google. Ask the right questions. For example:

- Lose weight naturally
- Lower blood sugar naturally
- Doctors that specialize in natural methods of healing and weight loss

When you hear people talk about who they follow or who helped them get their health back, connect with those names on Facebook, Instagram, LinkedIn, anywhere social. Follow them and learn from them. Yours truly does weekly training on

Facebook on these very topics, free.

Talk with friends and family who have lost weight, started working out, or changed their health naturally. Pick their brains. When people accomplish goals like this, they are happy to share the information.

If you take each section of this chapter and put it into practice each week or even each month, you will have accumulated life-changing, life-saving effects for your life. All while learning and enjoying the process.

Change is beautiful. Go be beautiful.

CHAPTER 10

YOU GOT THIS

You are strong, you are magnificent, you have got this!

"Give your dreams all you've got, and you'll be amazed at the energy that comes out of you."
—William James

Living with diabetes is hard.

Living with heart disease is hard.

Going through life overweight is hard.

Losing weight is simple, but it's not easy.

Getting your health under control is somewhat simple, but it's not easy. I say somewhat because it's more difficult to fix than it is to prevent.

There are multiple diseases that can be prevented and treated with nutrition. These are the ones that affected me and the ones I chose to specialize in.

Here's what I hope you've taken away from this book so far:

- If a disease or condition runs in your family, you're not necessarily destined or doomed to get it.
- Genetics is the roadmap for cellular breakdown, not a determination that you will have a certain disease or condition.
- If you eat right and move, you can prevent a lot of illness, disease, pain, and health obstacles in your life.
- You have the power to change your future and the future of generations that come after you.
- Even small steps, done consistently, can and will benefit you greatly.
- It's a marathon, not a sprint.
- Progress over perfection.

Have you ever known someone who has been thin since you met them, never seems to eat much, doesn't really like a lot of sugary things (you know that person, one cookie and they're done while you're watching to see if anyone notices you taking another), and always seems to be moving? You look at old photos, and even after giving birth they never seemed to hang on to any weight. Do you consider them lucky? Fortunate? Blessed? Think they just have great genes? Well, guess what? Most of that was learned behavior, most likely from their parents or family.

Many of us grew up being told to finish our meals whether we were full or not. If we did, we earned a sweet treat for doing so. Still not hungry but putting more food in. I'm not ripping on parents here, I had to finish meals too. But that teaches us to eat when we're not hungry. We're being trained to ignore our body's cues to stop.

Today, we live in a world where we can get our hands on any type of food almost anytime and anywhere. Post-COVID we can now have anything we want delivered right to our door. Our favorite gas stations produce their own food and have aisles full of snacks. I remember when a gas station barely had a selection of candy with a few choices of mints and gum. You can eat at these places three times a day if you want to now. In a hurry or out and about in bad weather? No problem, there's a drive-thru for that. We can even order on our phone.

The "easy button" is ruining our health. We grab something in a package and run out the door with our coffee. We have lunch with our office buddies or throw something into the microwave that came out of a box and has been frozen for who knows how long. Then we go home and maybe have time to make dinner or it's been in the crockpot, or we started the oven with our phone, but chances are, like many households, there are other things going on or we don't feel like cooking, so dinner is picked up at the drive-thru or restaurant or delivered to our door.

I've literally witnessed littles at a restaurant begging their parents to DoorDash food from a different restaurant, usually fast food, because they don't like the "big people food" at the restaurant they're at. That's just sad.

Folks, we don't have a genetics problem. We have a food problem.

"But I don't have time to cook."

According to Exploding Topics,[13] people spend an average of 2 hours and 24 minutes on social media every day.

---

[13] https://explodingtopics.com

Americans come in at 10 minutes less. According to Marketing Charts,[14] "During Q4 2022 the average US adult spent 294 minutes per day with TV." That's 4.9 hours. Surely there's some time there you can work with.

Meal prep is also a thing. People will prepare nutritious meals for you. They can cover your breakfast, lunch, and dinner. There are meal prep companies that make meals for families as well. Make sure these folks will sit down with you and go over menus and recipes. While it's nice that someone else is cooking, we're still responsible for knowing what's in our food.

"But I don't want to make separate meals for my kids or husband."

You may have to start small, but shouldn't your loved ones be eating well too? They are not exempt from our SAD (Standard American Diet) food when it comes to their health. They will eventually get on board.

"But I don't have time to exercise."

Refer to the information above about having time to cook. Perhaps social media time could be exchanged for playing a great playlist and going for a walk. Maybe a great podcast or an audio book would work for you. I'll tell you from personal experience, you can lift weights, march in place, or move in some way while you watch TV. I've done it, try it.

---

[14] https://marketingcharts.com

"But I don't like vegetables."

> One word, friends: Google! We live in a time in which information is literally at our fingertips. There are some vegetables that you like. Start there. Find recipes and play with them so that you can grow your options.

"My grocery store has a limited selection."

> Chances are there's a Whole Foods, Trader Joe's, Sprouts, or something similar near you. Maybe not, depending on where you live. Regardless, you may need to shop at multiple stores. There's this cool thing where you can order online and pick up. One of the few gifts to us from COVID. Use it. There are also grocery delivery companies out there. And, since we're going to eat better, let's put DoorDash, Instacart, and the others to work for us.

Now that we have some of the excuses out of the way, where does one start?

I'm going full-on coach with you here—please listen up. Only work on one to two things at a time. I'm not kidding. If you try to overhaul your entire life you will be miserable, overwhelmed, frustrated, and you won't stick with it. It took me years to get my health back. However, a silver lining for you: It only took about six to seven months to lose 26 pounds. Not bad.

Add the Water

Notice I didn't tell you to eliminate anything. Right now, we're going to add.

We can argue all day long about how much water to drink per day. If you're drinking less than 80 oz. of water per day, start with a 16.9 oz. bottle of water. Then build on that until you get to 80 oz. Or, find a formula that you are comfortable with, and shoot for that goal. Start small, work your way up to it. Yes, you will be in the bathroom more when you start. At some point your body will adjust and you won't have to go as often. I drink a gallon a day; I've done that for 30 years now and it just works for me. You do you, but drink your water. If you don't like plain water, look up water infusion recipes. I have some in the Guides section of my group which you can find at https://facebook.com/groups/ponytailgrit.

Add the Plants

Again, we're adding here. Again, there's argument as to how many servings you need. The range goes from five to nine servings per person per day. If you're not eating any fruits and vegetables, start with five. Work up from there. The closer you can eat them to natural, the better. Frozen is also good as the nutrients are still in the fruits or vegetables. In the beginning, just add them. Add them to every meal, use them for snacks. For anyone worried about spiking blood sugar with fruit, eat it at the end of a high protein meal or pair it with healthy fats like nut butter.

Add Movement

If you've done the first two items by now, you should be feeling better. Everyone's ability is going to be different. If you haven't exercised in years, you'll need to start with 5-10 minutes. I'm serious here and it's OK. Once you can do that, add five minutes each time until you're up to 45 minutes to an hour. Some days you'll be able to do more than others. It's OK. Some days you won't be able to do any at all. It's OK. If you miss a day jump back in. Missing a day is OK. Missing seven days is not, unless you're severely ill, in the hospital, etc. Find something that you like. If you don't, you won't stick with it. I dance, my husband punches a heavy bag. Find your thing!

Find other ways to move during sedentary parts of your day. A workout is great, but we need more than just that movement. Walk while you're on the phone, walk with other parents at your kid's practice, park at the back of the parking lot, take the stairs, bag your groceries in smaller bags and make multiple trips to the car. You are obviously excused from that during snow, ice, and thunderstorms. Walk your dog(s). Walk your cat(s). Play with your kids, your grandkids, or the neighbor's kids. Turn friend gatherings into game time outdoors when the weather allows. I'm talking frisbee, catch, or something active. Playing checkers outside doesn't count.

The goal is to get to 30 minutes or more of consistent activity for at least five days a week. As you shrink, you'll need to add more. Adding the additional activity to your day is a bonus and one your body and joints will thank you for.

Add Protein

Another one where there are multiple ways to get to the amount that you need. Find something you're comfortable with. I'm going to tell you right now that most of you will be shocked at how little protein you're eating. I was, and I'm a coach. Yes, that discovery happened well after I became a coach. Yes, that's a little embarrassing. We're human here.

Figure out what you think you need, then find out where you're at. If you don't want to do the research, I can recommend 80 grams of protein a day. You'll need to track your food for a bit. MyFitnessPal and Fitbit are great apps for that. There are others. Find one you like and will use and go for it.

Note: If you have heart disease markers you need to be careful here. Watch the red meat, use chicken and fish until you get to safer ground. I love red meat and I still eat it. I just don't eat it nearly as much as I used to. Vegetables, beans, and legumes also have protein in them.

Depending on where you're at with your health and weight, there's more to this. If you are diabetic, pre-diabetic, overweight, or have heart disease issues, these four basic things will change your life. If you've done these things and have arrived at a good spot, then you're ready to move on. Even if you don't need to lose weight, check and see where you're at with these things. I assure you, these four additions are life changing.

Add Accountability

You may or may not already know these things. Most of us have a good idea of how to lose weight. *But—you're not doing it!* This is where accountability comes in. Can you do this by yourself? You absolutely can! Will you do this by yourself? Chances are no, you won't. If you would and could, you wouldn't be reading this book.

Where can you find someone to help you with accountability?

Friends and Family

While this one seems like a great idea, be careful here. Your friends and family love you. They support you. They also want you to be happy. So, when the tough days come, they aren't holding up your "why" statement—they're not even thinking about it. They aren't going to be tough on you or hold you to the fire. They'll encourage you; they'll remind you of your goals, they'll try to help. They really will, and they mean well. But they don't want to risk hurting your feelings or making you feel bad. So, ultimately, if you push hard enough, they will cave. It's not their fault, they're human, like you. Some have absolutely utilized friends and family for accountability with success. Just know it's not the norm, and if it falls apart it's out of love and appreciation for the wonderful you.

Groups

This can be online, social media, or actual meet up in-person groups. Groups can be a little more effective because they don't know you as well as your beloved family and friends. You'll likely become friends too and hey, that's always cool! Plus, you all have similar goals, and it helps when you're not alone. Groups are most effective when there's a leader. A leader provides the group with someone to look up to, whether it's for starting the group or having blazed the trail before you. Having a leader provides an extra layer of accountability as we are tribal, and no one wants to let the leader down. Even without one, peer pressure can be a positive thing, and in this scenario it works well. Again, once they get to you know you, we're back to the "buddy" system. Another thing is that life happens, people quit coming, your friend isn't there anymore, and now you're missing meetings too. I created my group to build community and help with accountability. Some have had success just utilizing the group. You do you.

Coach

Remember coaches? Even if you didn't play sports, you likely ran into a coach during your school years. They were probably a gym teacher, or maybe they even taught one of your classes outside of the sports/fitness realm. I love coaches and wish I would have picked up on that many years ago. Did you slack in gym class? You sure didn't intentionally! Did you not turn in your homework in that class a coach taught? I sure had mine turned in! Did you chase butterflies on the ball field or court (OK–you know what I mean here) or did you get to work during practice? Did you work harder during a game? Um, yeah. Why? You didn't want to let them down.

When it comes to the sports setting you were under a coach because you desired to participate in a sport. Whether you had experience already or not, it's the coach's job to train the individual and create a team. If you Google "coach definition" (if you just Google "coach" you'll be looking at purses), it shows that a coach is a person who teaches and trains the members of a sports team and makes decisions about how the team plays during games. [15] It also says that coaches "provide an experience that helps clients move forward, feel at peace, achieve goals and become better versions of themselves." The latter is what I do. No whistle, no push-ups, no yelling, but I am here to get you where you want to be.

Coaches implement a group (team) and one-on-one skills with individual clients (players) to help people achieve what they knew to do but could not do on their own. That's why it's effective. You can hang with the group, you have your time with the coach, and months down the line you're like, "Wow, look at what I've done!" with that coach cheering you on more than any cheerleader on the planet. Do you need a coach to succeed at weight loss or improving your health? Not necessarily. Is it easier with a coach? You better believe it!

For the most part, I work with women because I am one. Health and weight loss is different for men and women. Gentlemen, I'm not opposed to working with you. I can and have in the past, so don't let my female marketing deter you from reaching out. I've also worked with married couples, which greatly helps with that issue of thinking that you have to make two meals.

If you've been on the internet for more than five minutes in your life, you know that there are literally thousands, possibly millions

---

[15] The Britannica Dictionary. "Coach."

of coaches. Life coaches, mindset coaches, business coaches, weight loss coaches, bikini competition coaches, weightlifting coaches, you name it. I have a coach! Not all coaches are the same, and you may need to search for a bit before you find one that you resonate with.

If you've enjoyed this book and think we might be a good match, you are welcome to join my group and participate in weekly live training free of charge. That way, you get a feel for who I am and what it's like to work with me. I also do free challenges throughout the year, which go a bit deeper than the training. If you feel that we are a good fit, I offer programs to help you lose weight, lower blood sugar, and get moving again. You may never work with me on a program, but you will have access to lots of great information and a wonderful group of people that have the same thing on their minds. And, if you don't think we're a good fit to work together but do feel like you would like to work with a coach, I'll help you find one. You just can't beat that.

In closing, I want you to know that you can take on anything and achieve your goals. You can live a healthy and active life, which is my heart's desire for you. Whether it's me, another coach, a group, or just you by yourself, you can absolutely do this. It's worth every tear, smile, drop of sweat, victory, and change that's made along the way.

Let's do this!

READY TO TAKE ACTION?
#HEALTHIEREVERYDAY
Lose Weight - Get Moving
With Ponytail Grit

Ponytail Grit was founded by Jeanna Crawford in September of 2020, when she answered the call to help busy women, like herself, lose weight and regain their health and vitality. Jeanna provides free, live weekly training with weight loss tips, nutrition instruction, and plenty of motivation to keep you going toward your goals. She also does free challenges in the group to provide you with hands-on learning for the life changes needed to put you on the right path. #Healthiereveryday represents that making small changes, one at a time, and building on those changes can create huge benefits for your health and well-being.

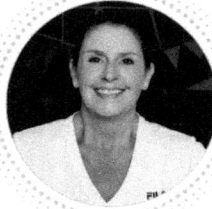

PONYTAIL GRIT

Helping busy women change
their shape, heal their body
and move again!

918.694.0211

https://facebook.com/groups/Ponytailgrit

Join Us in our Next Challenge

Ponytail Grit offers challenges to give you hands-on experience with coaching and healthy changes. Fitness challenges are also offered monthly.

For more information, visit us at
https://facebook.com/groups/ponytailgrit

Call or text: 918-694-0211

Email: Jeannalrich@gmail.com

ACKNOWLEDGMENTS

First, I'd like to thank God. For my health, for providing the knowledge I needed to get it back, and for the provisions already here to do just that.

I'd like to thank Dr. Chad Edwards at Revolution Health & Wellness for being a great doctor. He talks, listens, and cares. He and the other doctors and nurse practitioners were with me all the way. Thank you for being different. Thank you for truly caring.

I really appreciate my family for their support and understanding. There were some late nights, deadlines, and closed doors so that I could put this together. My husband, my son and his wife, my daughter, my dad and his wife, and my brother and sister-in-law all supported me in this. My grandbaby Millie added another layer to my vision of helping others. Thank you.

Special thanks to my business coach, Jessica Houligan, for not letting me stay in my comfort zone. While "progress over perfection" is something I have always believed in, without her I wouldn't have put that into practice as a coach and would still be waiting for "the perfect time" to get started. Because of that, I have happy clients and am ready to serve more.

Thank you to my clients for believing in me and allowing me to be part of your health journey. You don't know until you get into the actual coaching how this works, and their patience, attention, and enthusiasm keep me going every day.

Thank you to She Rises Studios, Michael Luna, Adriana Luna Carlos, Catherine Cruz, Sarah Salting, and Parker Shatkin for the opportunity, guidance and support. This wouldn't have come together without them. Ladies, if you have a story to tell, get connected with She Rises Studios, they will help you.

This may seem odd, but I'd also like to thank myself. For getting way out of my comfort zone, committing to this, and seeing it through. For sharing a story that makes me feel vulnerable, but I know will help others down the road.

ABOUT THE AUTHOR

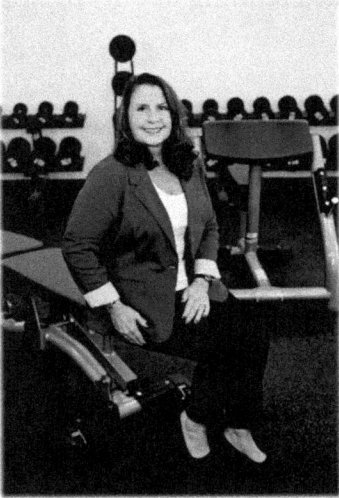

I'm Jeanna Crawford, an Okie since birth, wife, mother, grandmother, daughter, sister, aunt, niece and granddaughter. I'm also a nutrition coach and Zumba fitness instructor.

It breaks my heart to see ladies struggle with their health and their weight. I was one of those ladies myself.

One day in my doctor's office I was told that I was prediabetic, inflamed, and my heart disease markers were in a bad place. My joints hurt, the movement was painful, I got winded easily, and I could hardly bend over to tie my shoes. For someone who's always been active, this was not a happy time in my life. Fortunately, I have a great doctor and we discussed how I could back out of this without being on traditional medications. Soon after, going through my mom's things after her passing, I found a book about healing with nutrition.

I became obsessed and enrolled in a nutrition certification program. I practiced what I learned, found a way to move again (thank you Zumba), lost 26 pounds, and with some time and effort, regained my health.

I want to help you do the same!

When I'm not coaching or dancing I enjoy being on a motorcycle with my husband, playing with our pups, playing with the grandbaby, or hanging out in the backyard tending to our tropical plants.

https://www.facebook.com/jeanna.h.richards
https://www.facebook.com/groups/ponytailgrit
https://www.facebook.com/PonytailGrit
https://ponytailgrit.com
https://www.instagram.com/jea3296/
https://www.instagram.com/ponytailgrit/

www.ingramcontent.com/pod-product-compliance
Lightning Source LLC
Chambersburg PA
CBHW060245030426

42335CB00014B/1606